INTRODUCTION TO ELECTROCARDIOGRAPHY

D1548179

INTRODUCTION TO
ELECTROCARDIOGRAPHY

SECOND EDITION

J. WILLIS HURST, M.D.

Professor and Chairman, Department of Medicine
Emory University School of Medicine and Hospitals
Atlanta, Georgia

ROBERT J. MYERBURG, M.D.

Associate Professor of Medicine and Assistant
Professor of Physiology, University of Miami School of Medicine
Chief, Cardiology Section, Veterans Administration Hospital
Miami, Florida

McGRAW-HILL BOOK COMPANY
A Blakiston Publication

New York   St. Louis   San Francisco   Düsseldorf   Johannesburg
Kuala Lumpur   London   Mexico   Montreal   New Delhi   Panama
Rio de Janeiro   Singapore   Sydney   Toronto

INTRODUCTION TO ELECTROCARDIOGRAPHY

1 2 3 4 5 6 7 8 9 0 H D B P 7 9 8 7 6 5 4 3

This book was set in Caledonia by Monotype Composition Company, Inc. The editors were Paul K. Schneider and Ida Abrams Wolfson; the designer was Nicholas Krenitsky; and the production supervisor was Sally Ellyson.
The printer was Halliday Lithograph Corporation; the binder, The Book Press, Inc.

Library of Congress Cataloging in Publication Data

Hurst, John Willis, 1920–
    Introduction to electrocardiography.

    "A Blakiston publication."
    "The first nine chapters . . . were published in 1952
. . . [under title:] Atlas of spatial vector
electrocardiography [by J. W. Hurst and G. C. Woodson]"
    Bibliography: p.
    1. Vectorcardiography. I. Myerburg, Robert J.,
joint author. II. Hurst, John Willis, 1920–
Atlas of spatial vector electrocardiography.
III. Title. [DNLM: 1. Electrocardiography. WG 140
H966i 1973]
RC683.5.V4H87   1973   616.1'2'0754   73-1683

ISBN 0-07-031464-0

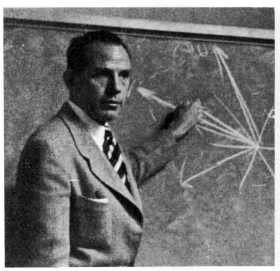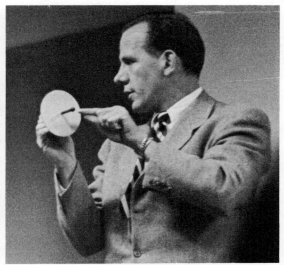

DR. ROBERT P. GRANT—TEACHING*

This book is dedicated to the memory of Dr. Robert P. Grant—a unique individual who influenced a vast number of medical students, house officers, and colleagues with his brilliant, creative mind and his warm and kind personality.

* Photographs of Dr. Robert P. Grant made at Emory University in 1954 by Dr. Leslie French of Hyattsville, Maryland. Dr. Grant developed the spatial vector method of analyzing electrocardiograms while he was a member of the Department of Medicine of Emory University School of Medicine (1947–1950).

CONTENTS

Left Ventricular Hypertrophy

Direction of the mean and instantaneous spatial QRS vectors; magnitude of the QRS complexes; duration of the QRS complexes; direction of the mean spatial T vector; direction of the mean spatial ST vector.

PART TWO. THE CARDIAC ARRHYTHMIAS

PREFACE

The field of electrocardiography has changed in two ways. (1) Ten years ago only a few physicians "interpreted" the graphs, but now it is different. Numerous physicians and many nurses and allied health personnel have become quite proficient in "interpreting" electrocardiograms. (2) More recently—during the last 5 years—the scientific discoveries of a few men have made their way to the area of practical electrocardiography. Witness the new views about conduction disturbances in the atria and ventricles (see Chapter 5). Except for Chapter 5, the content of this book, however, has been changed very little. We have not made alterations in the text of this edition except where a practical implication is clearly seen. In this way we have maintained the simplicity and admitted dogma of the forerunners of this edition.

This book is divided into two parts. Each part presents a teaching concept.

PART ONE. The first nine chapters of this part deal almost exclusively with that portion of the electrocardiogram that is produced by the ventricular myocardium. This includes the QRS complex, ST segment, and T wave. Chapter 10 covers the analysis of the P wave (atrial activity). *The aim of this portion of the book is to teach the vector concept and to show how the concept can be applied to each and every tracing.* The first nine chapters of the book were published in 1952. The principles of the vector concept have not changed, and the material presented in 1952 is as useful in teaching now as it was then. Dr. Gratton Woodson, a coauthor of the book *Atlas of Spatial Vector Electrocardiography*, could not join us in the later editions because of his commitments to the practice of medicine. The following excerpt from the preface of the *Atlas* is reproduced here:

Three methods are available for studying the electrical forces of the heart. Each of the methods has limitations, advantages, and disadvantages. When a pattern method of interpretation is used, one memorizes deflection contours and by experience knows whether the pattern is within normal limits or resembles a specific pattern previously found to be abnormal. The same electrocardiographic leads and deflections used in the pattern method are utilized in spatial vector electrocardiography. In the latter method, the direction of the electrical forces responsible for the electrocardiographic waves are visualized in space and are represented as vectors. Vectorcardiography, on the other hand, uses different equipment and different electrode attachments. This method, utilizing an oscilloscope, actually records the directions and magnitude of the instantaneous electrical forces of the heart and allows one to study the P, QRS, ST, and T loops. By using proper electrode attachments one can obtain several views of the underlying electrical forces and the spatial loops can be visualized. This monograph deals almost exclusively with vector electrocardiography.

Vector electrocardiography offers certain advantages over the conventional pattern method. (1) Most textbooks explain the theoretical aspects of electrocardiography by using vector principles but then make no use of such principles in explaining electrocardiograms in clinical practice. In the vector method of interpretation, basic vector principles are used in practice as well as in theory. (2) The deflections recorded in twelve routine leads can be illustrated by two or more spatial vectors and the details of deflection contour need not be memorized. (3) When vector principles are utilized in interpreting an electrocardiogram, one is able to offer reasonable explanations for unusual or previously unexplained tracings. (4) In our experience vector electrocardiography has no peer in stimulating interest in medical students, and, therefore, the vector method is a useful tool. Indeed, it was the value of a new and effective method of teaching which prompted us to complete this manuscript. (5) Electrocardiographic patterns are automatically learned as one is learning to plot the direction of various electrical forces of the heart and a pattern learned by such a method has a rational explanation for its origin.

The basic concepts of the spatial vector method of electrocardiography are diagrammatically illustrated and discussed. Many of the diagrams will seem oversimplified. Often we have sacrificed complete accuracy in our endeavor to present facts in their most elementary and useful form. This will no doubt embarrass, offend, and emotionally disturb the scientist who is an expert in physics, electricity, or electrocardiography. We offer no apologies for the liberties we have taken since we feel justified in sacrificing exactness in our effort to explain the complicated electrical activity of the heart. No claims are made that the directions of the spatial vectors determined by the method discussed indicate the true directions of the electrical forces of the heart. Indeed, so many obvious simplifications are made that we are certain that such is not the case. For instance, the electrical forces of the heart are treated as though they arise in the exact center of the chest of every subject. The chest is represented as a cylinder and is assumed to be a homogeneous volume conductor. The chest lead electrode positions are drawn on the cylindrical replica of the chest at fixed points whereas in reality the electrode positions vary from subject to subject. The transitional pathways for various vectors are illustrated as the edge of a disk. Actually, the transitional pathway is more irregular than is indicated, especially when the chest is of small size. Despite these simplifications, however, the vector method of electrocardiography can be utilized in routine practice because there is no doubt that the method is sufficiently accurate for clinical work.

Our interest in vector electrocardiography began with our association with Dr. Robert Grant and Dr. Harvey Estes in the Department of Cardiology at Emory University Medical School in 1949. The present monograph could not have been written without their very excellent basic work. In 1951, the Blakiston Company published *Spatial Vector Electrocardiography*, written by Grant and Estes. The present monograph is an extension of the Grant and Estes material to include the clinical application of the vector method. We sincerely thank Dr. Grant for his constant help and guidance during the preparation of this manuscript.

PART TWO. The second portion of the book deals with the electrocardiographic presentation of cardiac arrhythmias. *The purpose of this portion is to teach by the use of the A-V diagram or ladder.* The electrocardiographic presentation of cardiac arrhythmias should not be memorized any more than that of the ventricular electrocardiogram (QRS-T) should be. Accordingly, the use of the A-V diagram as a method of teaching is presented with the hope that a more basic understanding of arrhythmias can be introduced to the beginner.

The authors did not originate either the spatial vector method of interpreting the ventricular electrocardiogram or the use of the A-V ladder to teach arrhythmias. Dr. Robert Grant, working in the Department of Medicine at Emory University School of Medicine at Grady Memorial Hospital, deserves the credit for introducing the method known as *spatial vector electrocardiography*. Sir Thomas Lewis, working in London, deserves the credit for introducing the A-V ladder. We have attempted to simplify the two teaching methods in order to present them to a wider audience.

An appendix of tables and a glossary are included in order to clarify the subject matter. A bibliography (including journals and books) is also included so that an interested student can be guided into the voluminous world of electrocardiographic literature.

We wish to thank Grover Hogan, Patsy Bryan, Bob Beveridge, and Eddie Jackson for their efforts in creating diagrams that matched the illustrations of earlier editions. We are deeply indebted to Carol Miller of the Department of Medicine, Emory University School of Medicine, and Joyce Freeman for their assistance in preparing the new manuscript and to Paul Schneider of McGraw-Hill for his assistance in publishing "Introduction to Electrocardiography."

J. WILLIS HURST
ROBERT J. MYERBURG

INTRODUCTION TO ELECTROCARDIOGRAPHY

PART ONE

The Spatial Vector Method and Its Clinical Application

CHAPTER ONE

The Spatial Vector Method

The Definition of An Electrocardiogram. A small amount of electrical energy is generated by the heart during each cardiac cycle. This electrical energy, or force, is picked up and greatly amplified by the electrocardiographic machine and recorded on a strip of moving paper. It is this record that is termed an electrocardiogram. These events are illustrated in fig. 1.

Definitions of the Various Electrocardiographic Waves and Intervals. The record consists of a series of waves which were originally labeled, purely arbitrarily by Einthoven, the P wave, the QRS complex, the T wave, and the U wave (fig. 2).

The P Wave. The P wave is produced by the spread of the electrical activity through the atrial musculature.

The QRS Complex. The QRS complex is produced by the spread of the electrical activity through the ventricular musculature. This process, resulting in the loss of electrical charges, is termed depolarization.

The Q Wave. The Q wave is the first downward deflection of the QRS complex preceding the R wave.

The R Wave. The R wave is the first upward deflection of the QRS complex.

The S Wave. The S wave is the first downward deflection of the QRS complex which follows the R wave.

The R' Wave. The R' wave is the second upward deflection of the QRS complex.

A QS Complex. A QS complex implies that the entire ventricular complex is downward and the Q wave and the S wave are "fused."

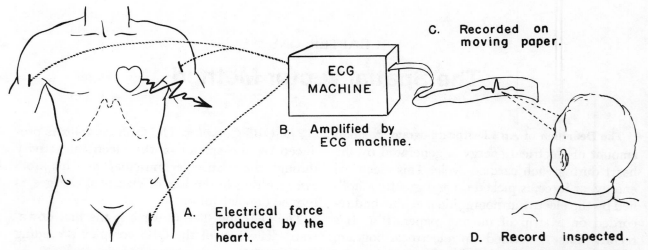

FIG. 1. Electrical forces of the heart are amplified and recorded on moving paper to produce the electrocardiogram.

The T Wave. The T wave is produced when the ventricles rebuild the electrical charges which were lost as the QRS complex was produced. This process is termed repolarization.

The U Wave. The U wave follows the T wave and is sometimes of clinical significance.

The P-Q or P-R Interval. The P-Q interval, or P-R interval if there is no Q wave, represents the time required for the electrical impulse to pass through the atrial musculature plus the delay of that impulse at the atrioventricular node. The P-Q interval in the normal person varies with

4

age and heart rate. (See Table 1 in Appendix.) The P-Q interval is measured from the beginning of the P wave to the beginning of the Q wave. When no Q wave is present, the P-R interval is measured from the beginning of the P wave to the beginning of the R wave.

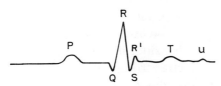

FIG. 2. The deflections of an electrocardiogram.

The QRS Interval. The duration of the QRS interval is measured from the beginning of the first wave of the QRS complex to the end of the last wave and should not exceed .10 second in the normal adult.

The Q-T Interval. The Q-T interval is measured from the beginning of the QRS complex to the end of the T wave. It varies with heart rate, age, and sex. The upper limits of normal are shown in the Appendix (Table 2).

The ST Segment. The ST segment is that portion of the electrocardiogram between the end of the QRS complex and the beginning of the T wave.

The P wave, QRS complex, T wave, and U waves are recorded on special paper having time markings and amplitude lines. The smaller squares are 1 millimeter square and their sides represent .1 millivolt. For convenience, every fifth vertical and horizontal line is made slightly heavier so that one large square thus formed indicates .2 second duration along the horizontal side and .5 millivolt amplitude along the vertical side (fig. 3). All electrocardiograms are standardized so that 1 millivolt of electrical force will move the recording stylus or string 10 millimeters.

The Approach to the Electrocardiogram. The portion of the electrocardiogram produced by the ventricular musculature, namely the QRS, ST, and T deflections, can be interpreted by two methods.

1. The physician can study the contours of the deflections in the electrocardiograms of

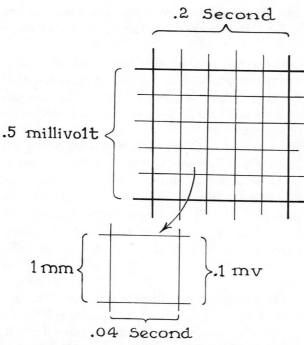

.2 Second

.5 millivolt

1 mm

.1 mv

.04 Second

Fig. 3. Diagram showing the special time markings and amplitude lines found on electrocardiographic paper.

numerous normal individuals and establish the normal range. He then assumes that any deviation from the normal range is abnormal. By associating heart abnormalities with their corresponding abnormal electrocardiograms, he learns that various cardiac lesions are associated with certain electrocardiographic "patterns." For example, if a patient with a clinical history or pathologic proof of a myocardial infarction has a specific type of electrocardiogram, it would be logical to consider myocardial infarction each time that electrocardiographic pattern appeared. This conventional method of analysis is called pattern interpretation.

This is an excellent method of analysis but unfortunately it requires a great deal of memorization since the normal range is wide and there may be only minor differences between many of the abnormal electrocardiograms. This method, requiring detailed description, corresponds to a verbal description of the physical appearance of a criminal; for example, 6 feet tall, blue eyes, scar on left cheek, and tattoo on left forearm.

2. In the second method of interpretation, the physician inspects the electrocardiogram and

visualizes the electrical force which produces it. Abnormalities are recognized as abnormalities of direction or magnitude of the electrical forces or their relationship to each other.

In this method, now called the vector method of interpretation, a "picture" of the electrical force itself is produced. This method would correspond to a photograph of a criminal rather than a word description.

There is no question that the pattern method of interpretation is satisfactory. After all, we recognize our friends from day to day by being able to remember their appearance. Even a verbal description of individuals not as familiar to us as our friends will suffice if the description is good enough and the number of persons described is small. There are certain advantages of the vector method over the pattern method, just as a photograph of a person may give more information than a description. It is a more basic approach to electrocardiography, offering tools for the study of tracings one will encounter which have not been previously explained. It requires less memory work since the details of wave form occurring in the numerous leads need not be memorized.

The Electrical Forces of the Heart. Before considering the electrocardiogram, it is necessary to illustrate certain aspects of the electrical field which produces it. The presence of an electrical force originating at the center of a conducting medium, such as the human chest, sets up lines of electrical potential throughout the medium. To illustrate this, the human chest is depicted as a large cylinder. A frontal plane view, or cross section, of an electrical field produced by an electrical force whose origin is centrally located in a cylinder is shown in fig. 4.

The electrical field is much more intense immediately around the origin of the force which is represented by an arrow. The field has two halves, a negative and a positive half. The circles represent lines of equipotentiality and, as indicated by larger and larger "rings," the potential decreases as the distance from the origin of electrical force increases. Separating the negative (−) and positive (+) halves of the electrical field is a region which is at zero potential. The region of zero potential is always perpendicular to the direction of the electrical force. If the force changes in direction, the region of

7

zero potential and the negative and positive halves of the field also change.

Thus far, only a frontal plane view or cross section of an electrical field has been shown.

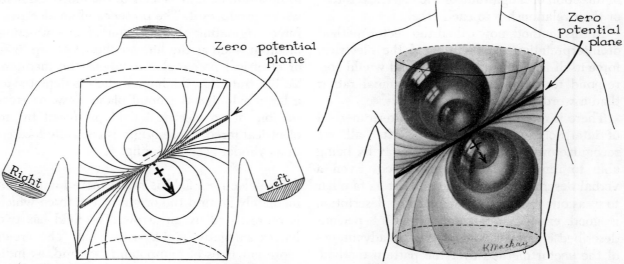

FIG. 4. A frontal plane view of an electrical field. The origin of the electrical force is located at the center of the cylinder. Note the region of zero potential separating the positive and negative halves of the electrical field. The region of zero potential is perpendicular to the direction of electrical force. The rings represent lines of equipotentiality. For simplicity only three rings are shown. This schematic illustration is not intended to show all the details of an electrical field.

FIG. 5. A diagrammatic illustration of an electrical field in three-dimensional space. The lines of equipotential are illustrated as spheres or shells. For simplicity only three shells are completed. The region, or plane, of zero potential is perpendicular to the direction of electrical force and extends in all directions to intersect the surface of the cylinder. This simple diagram is not intended to represent all that is known about an electrical field.

It should be obvious that the lines of equipotential are not simply rings as shown in the preceding diagram but are shells, or spheres (fig. 5). The shells extend in *all directions* to intersect the surface of the cylinder or chest, indicating that an electrical field is a three-dimensional figure. The region of zero potential always remains perpendicular to the direction of the electrical force and extends in all directions to intersect the surface of the cylinder, producing the transitional pathway which will be described in detail later.

The preceding discussion and the illustrations have been concerned with the effect of a single electrical force. Actually an electrocardiogram is produced by an infinite number of electrical forces occurring in a sequence and is therefore a great deal more complicated than the preceding discussion indicates.

The Electrical Forces of the Heart Represented by Vectors. Any force, be it mechanical or electrical, that has magnitude, direction, and sense can be considered as a vector and represented by an arrow. We see examples of mechanical force daily and it is useful to represent a familiar force by an arrow. For example, suppose a piece of meat is weighed with a pair of spring scales (fig. 6A). The weight is 4 pounds and the weight exerts its effect straight downward. An arrow can be drawn to illustrate the mechanical force produced by the 4 pounds of weight. The length of the arrow could indicate the amount of the weight, its direction could indicate the direction along which the force is exerted, and the arrowhead could indicate the "sense" of the force. In fig. 6B a vector is used to represent the mechanical force shown in fig. 6A.

Note that the arrow shaft is given a length of four units. If the same basic units are used to illustrate a weight of 8 pounds, then the arrow would be drawn twice as long (fig. 6C and fig. 6D).

The electrical forces of the heart have magnitude, direction, and sense and can, therefore, be considered as vectors and represented on paper by arrows.

As the excitation wave proceeds through the ventricular myocardium, electrical forces which are generated vary in magnitude and direction from instant to instant during a single QRS cycle. This variation in magnitude and direction

9

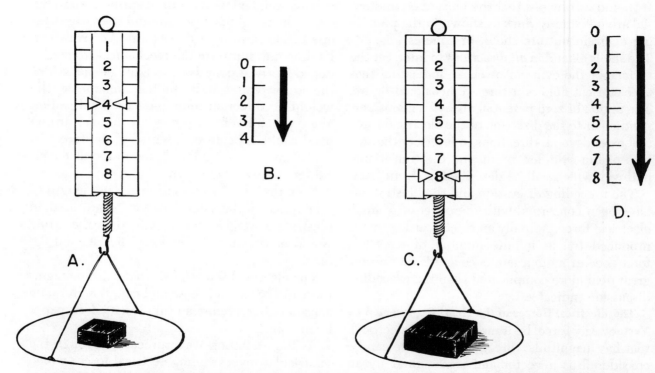

FIG. 6. Mechanical force represented as a vector. **(A)** Scales with a 4-lb. weight. **(B)** Arrow divided into four units directed downward. **(C)** Scales with an 8-lb. weight. **(D)** Arrow divided into eight units directed downward.

of electrical forces is due to the characteristic distribution of the conduction system and the varying thickness of the ventricular muscle.

This is illustrated very schematically by the seven vectors shown in fig. 7A. Actually each of the vectors shown represents magnitude and direction at successive instants and each of these is the summation of an infinite number of vectors generated from all points being excited at that given instant.

These instantaneous vectors can be treated as if they arise from a common origin at the relative zero point of the electrical field since the origins of the individual vectors are electrically

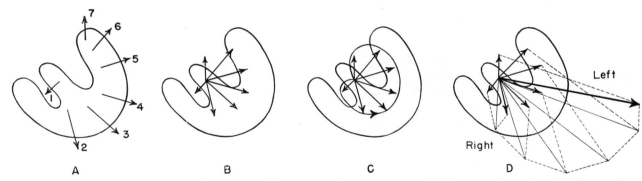

A　　　　B　　　　C　　　　D

Fig. 7. Diagram illustrating depolarization of the ventricular musculature as viewed in the frontal plane. (A) The numbered arrows indicate the sequence in which instantaneous electrical forces are generated during a single QRS cycle. (B) The instantaneous electrical forces, or vectors, drawn as if all forces arise at a common origin. (C) A line drawn through the termini of the instantaneous vectors produce the QRS loop. (D) The mean QRS vector is produced by vector summation of the instantaneous forces. Vector summation is accomplished by constructing a parallelogram using two vectors for its sides. The diagonal of the parallelogram will represent the vector sum for the two vectors.

11

relatively equidistant from the recording electrodes (fig. 7B).

It can be seen that each QRS deflection is due to a great number of instantaneous electrical forces or vectors. If a line is drawn through the termini of all the instantaneous vectors, a "loop" will be formed which reflects the change in magnitude and direction of vectors from instant to instant in a single cycle. When only the vectors generated during the QRS cycle are depicted, it is called a QRS loop (fig. 7C). When all the instantaneous vectors are added together, the resultant is termed the mean QRS. The mean QRS represents the average direction and magnitude of all the instantaneous QRS vectors (fig. 7D).

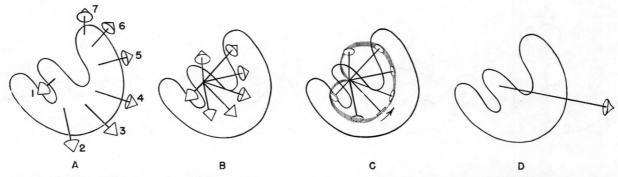

A   B   C   D

FIG. 8. Diagram illustrating depolarization of the ventricular musculature as viewed in space. (A) The numbered arrows indicate the sequence in which electrical forces are generated during a single QRS cycle, drawn in three-dimensional space (i.e., vector No. 1 not only is directed to the right and downward but also is directed slightly anteriorly and vector No. 7 is directed upward and posteriorly). (B) The spatial instantaneous forces, or vectors, illustrated as if all forces arise at a common origin. (C) A line drawn through the termini of the spatial instantaneous vectors produce the spatial QRS loop. (D) The mean spatial QRS vector is the net effective vector of all the spatial instantaneous vectors.

Thus far, the QRS vectors have been drawn as if the electrical forces occurred in only one plane. Since the ventricular portion of the heart is roughly hemispherical, the electrical forces may be directed in an anterior or a posterior direction, as well as in a horizontal or vertical direction. This orientation in space is indicated in fig. 8A, B, C, D by the tilt of the arrow's tip.

The preceding discussion has dealt only with the QRS forces but similar basic principles apply when the T forces are considered.

How to Measure the Electrical Forces of the Heart. The instrument used to measure electrical potential is the galvanometer. This instrument consists of a "volt-measuring dial" between two lead wires. One lead wire is attached to the positive side or pole of the galvanometer while the other wire is connected to the negative pole of the galvanometer and the difference in potential between the two lead wires is indicated by the position of the needle on the dial (fig. 9).

The modern electrocardiograph machine is simply a highly sensitive type of galvanometer. The basic galvanometric part of the instrument

has been modified in several ways so that the electrical forces of the heart can be measured with ease. (1) The modern electrocardiograph machine enables one to record moment-to-moment variation in the electrical forces by having the galvanometer's measuring "needle" write on a strip of moving paper. (2) A switch box allows one to change from one group of electrode

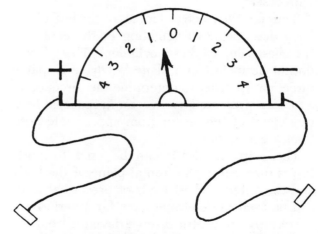

FIG. 9. Diagrammatic illustration of a galvanometer. Note the positive and negative poles and the "volt-measuring dial" between them.

positions to another quickly without having to attach and unattach the lead wires. Although this is convenient it frequently obscures the true wire connections which are used for a particular lead. Such wire connections must be memorized since they have been established by convention. (3) The lead wires can be connected to electrodes which can be attached to the patient with ease.

Thus far, the electrical forces of the heart have been described as originating in the center of the chest (depicted as a cylinder). These forces do not lie in just one plane but have a spatial direction. In order to determine the direction of a force, represented by a vector in space, at least two views of the vector from appropriate positions are necessary.

The extremity leads can be used to study forces directed in the frontal plane of the body and the anterior chest leads or precordial leads can be used to determine how far anteriorly or posteriorly an electrical force deviates from the frontal plane. These leads will now be described in detail.

The Extremity Leads. Einthoven first defined the galvanometric connections of Leads I, II, III. He assumed that electrodes placed on the left arm, right arm, and one leg are electrically if not anatomically equidistant from the origin of electrical force generated by the heart. A line through the body connecting the two points where the negative and positive poles of the galvanometer have been attached to the lead wires is called a lead axis. Hence, if the electrode positions of Leads I, II, III are electrically equidistant from the origin of electrical force, the lead axes produced by such electrodes would form the sides of an equilateral triangle (fig. 10A). The term equilateral in this case refers to an "electrically equilateral triangle" and not an "anatomically equilateral triangle." By translating the sides of the triangle to a common central point, Bayley has constructed a triaxial reference system. The axes of this figure are 60° apart (fig. 10B). By Einthoven's convention, the negative pole of the galvanometer is attached to the right arm and the positive pole of the galvanometer is attached to the left arm to record Lead I; the negative pole of the galvanometer is attached to the right arm and the positive pole of the galvanometer is attached to the left leg to record Lead II, and the negative pole is attached to the left arm and the positive pole to the left leg to record Lead III. *This must be memorized since it is a purely arbitrary arrangement.* When an electrical force is directed toward the electrode connected to the positive pole of the galvanometer an upright, or positive, deflection will be recorded and when an electrical force is directed away from the electrode connected to the positive pole of the galvanometer a downward, or negative, deflection will be recorded. The magnitude of deflection on Lead I plus the magnitude of deflection on Lead III equals the mag-

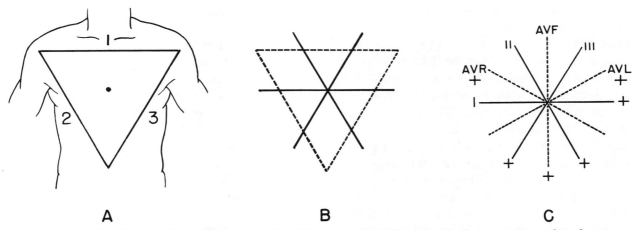

Fig. 10. (A) The "electrical" equilateral triangle of Einthoven. (B) The triaxial reference system of Bayley is produced when the sides of the Einthoven triangle are translated to a common central point. (C) The hexaxial reference system is produced by combining the triaxial system of Bayley with the unipolar extremity lead axes.

15

nitude of deflection on Lead II. This equation has a great deal of practical value, as will be emphasized later. These leads are termed bipolar leads since both lead wires of the galvanometer are introduced into the electrical field and the galvanometer records the difference in electrical potential influencing the ends of the wires.

Wilson later introduced "unipolar" extremity leads. In this system, the positive pole of the galvanometer is attached in turn to the right arm, left arm, and left leg while the negative pole is attached to a terminal at relative zero potential in the frontal plane achieved by interconnections to the three extremities. This terminal approaches zero potential since in such a network the potential of the right arm (VR) plus the potential at the left arm (VL) plus the potential at the left leg (VF) will equal zero. When drawn on the Einthoven graph of the three bipolar leads, the axes of the unipolar leads pass from the corners of the Einthoven triangle to the origin of electrical force located in the center of the triangle. These extremity lead axes will bisect the 60° angles of the tri-

axial system. Larger deflections are recorded by the technique of Goldberger without materially affecting the potential of the central terminal. Such leads are then called augmented unipolar extremity leads and are identified by the symbols aV_R, aV_L, and aV_F. The unipolar leads are so termed because only the positive pole of the galvanometer, the exploring electrode, is introduced into the electrical field of the heart, while the negative pole is attached to a point of zero potential. The difference in electrical potential is again recorded, but in this case, since one pole is at zero potential, the tracing is exclusively a recording of potential at the location on the body where the electrode is attached to the positive pole of the galvanometer. The augmented unipolar extremity leads will be used throughout this book.

If the axes of the unipolar and bipolar extremity leads are superimposed, a reference figure with six axes is obtained. This figure should logically be called the hexaxial reference system (fig. 10C). The polarity of the six extremity leads is indicated by a plus sign at the positive side of the lead axis and, although not indicated, the opposite side of the lead axis is negative.

16

Certain aspects of the hexaxial reference system deserve additional comment. A lead axis in the bipolar system is perpendicular to one of the unipolar extremity lead axes. More specifically, Lead axis aV_F is perpendicular to Lead axis I, aV_L is perpendicular to II, and aV_R is perpendicular to III. The magnitude of deflection on the augmented unipolar extremity leads is less than the magnitude of deflection on the bipolar extremity leads, but this is no drawback, since in the method for electrocardiographic interpretation being described, we are primarily concerned with the direction rather than the magnitude of the electrical force.

The bipolar and unipolar extremity leads are frequently called frontal plane leads because their lead axes lie in the frontal plane of body. These leads are considered to be spatial leads. In other words, the extremity electrodes are remote enough from the origin of electrical force to record equivalently from all parts of the heart. The contours of the unipolar extremity lead deflections differ from those of the bipolar extremity leads only because the lead axes have a different direction in the electrical field. In the vector method the unipolar and bipolar extremity leads are given equal value and are used only to determine the direction of the various electrical forces under study, six axes being more accurate than three.

The Influence of the Electrical Forces on the Extremity Leads. Having described the lead axes for the frontal plane of the body it is now necessary to show how electrical forces are projected on these leads. In order to understand the principle of projection it is useful to illustrate the concept with a diagram dealing with familiar objects. In fig. 11 a rod is placed between a light source and a screen. When the light is turned on, a shadow is projected on the screen. In such an illustration the screen is analogous to a lead axis and the rod corresponds to an electrical force. The shadow cast on the screen will be smallest when the rod is perpendicular to the screen (fig. 11A). The shadow cast on the screen will be largest when the rod is parallel with the screen (fig. 11B). There is a striking similarity between this simple example and the projection of electrical force on a lead axis. In fig. 12 a vector, representing an electrical force, is drawn perpendicular to a lead axis and no deflection is obtained, but when the vector is parallel to the

17

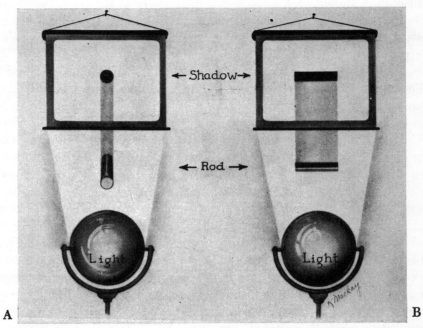

Fig. 11. Diagram illustrating the principle of projection, utilizing a light source, rod, and screen. (A) The light strikes the rod so that a shadow is cast on the screen. In this case the rod is perpendicular to the screen and the shadow is very small. The screen is analogous to a lead axis and the rod corresponds to a vector. (B) The light strikes the rod so that a shadow is cast on the screen. In this case the rod is parallel with the screen and the shadow cast is quite large. One should actually perform such an experiment with a pencil placed near the screen and the light source placed at a distance.

lead axis, its largest deflection will be recorded. If the vector is located somewhere between these two extremes, the magnitude of the deflection will be determined by how much the vector impinges or is projected on the lead axis. The amount of impingement is determined by drawing a line from the end of the vector to and perpendicular with the lead axis.

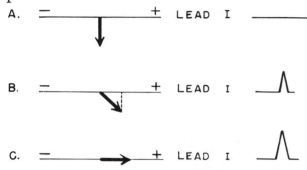

FIG. 12. (A) An electrical force illustrated as a vector, perpendicular to a given lead axis will record no deflection on that lead. (B) An electrical force, illustrated as a vector, located somewhere between the extremes illustrated in (A) and (C) will have a deflection magnitude equal to the amount that the vector impinges or is projected on that particular lead axis. (C) An electrical force, illustrated as a vector, parallel to a given lead axis will record its largest deflection on that lead.

The diagrams shown in figs. 11 and 12 illustrate a very basic and important principle of the vector method; namely, that when an electrical force is directed relatively perpendicular to a given lead axis, the smallest deflection will be recorded in that lead and when an electrical force is directed relatively parallel with a given lead axis, the largest deflection will be recorded in that lead. In fig. 13A a vector, representing an electrical force, is directed slightly downward and to the left. When the hexaxial reference system is superimposed on such a figure it can be seen that the vector is perpendicular to the Lead III axis (fig. 13B). Accordingly, the smallest extremity lead deflection will be recorded in Lead III. Stated another way, when the smallest extremity lead deflection is found in Lead III, the vector representing that deflection must be relatively perpendicular to Lead III. In fig. 14A a vector, representing an electrical force, is directed downward and to the left. When the hexaxial reference system is superimposed on such a figure it can be seen that the vector is parallel with Lead II (fig. 14B). Accordingly, the largest extremity lead deflection

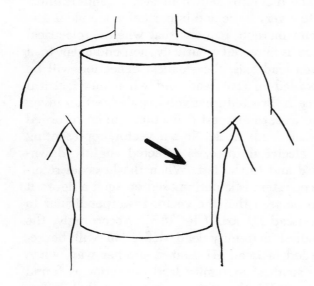

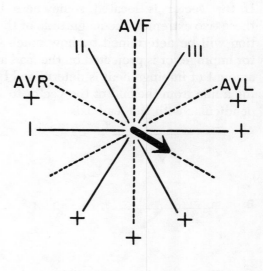

A.

B.

Fig. 13. (A) An electrical force represented by a vector located in the center of the chest. (B) The hexaxial reference system superimposed on the vector. One can determine the degree of positivity or negativity of the extremity leads by drawing a line from the tip of the arrow head to and perpendicular with each of the lead axes. The vector is perpendicular to Lead III and therefore the vector does not project on that lead. Accordingly, Lead III records no deflection. Leads I and II are equally positive, Lead aV_R is large and negative, and Leads aV_L and aV_F are equally positive.

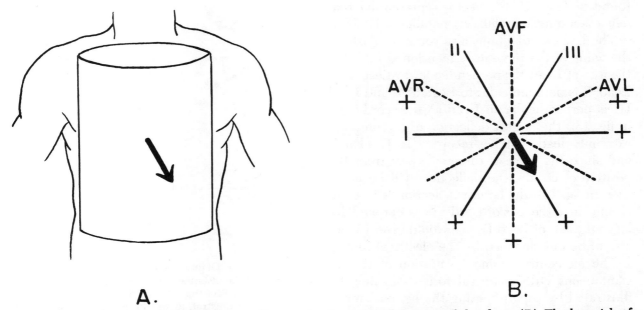

A.

B.

FIG. 14. (A) An electrical force represented by a vector located in the center of the chest. (B) The hexaxial reference system superimposed on the vector. Lead II records the largest deflection because the vector projects its greatest amount on that lead. Leads I and III are equally positive. Lead aV$_L$ is uninfluenced by the electrical field because the vector is perpendicular to it. Lead aV$_R$ is negative, and aV$_F$ is similar in size but is positive.

will be found in Lead II. Stated in another way, when the largest extremity lead deflection is found in Lead II, the vector representing that deflection must be relatively parallel to Lead II.

The last two diagrams also serve to illustrate the value of the previously mentioned fact that the axis of Lead I is perpendicular to Lead aV$_F$, Lead II is perpendicular to Lead aV$_L$, and Lead III is perpendicular to Lead aV$_R$. Accordingly, in fig. 13B the largest deflection of the unipolar extremity leads will be recorded in Lead aV$_R$ and since the force is directed away from the positive electrode, the deflection will be negative. In fig. 14B the largest deflection is in Lead II and since the axis of Lead aV$_L$ is perpendicular to the axis of Lead II, one would expect Lead aV$_L$ to be uninfluenced by the electrical force.

The moment-to-moment variation of the instantaneous QRS electrical forces can now be illustrated by superimposing the hexaxial reference system on the instantaneous QRS vectors and drawing lines from the termini of these vectors to and perpendicular with a given lead axis. In this way one can see how an electrocardiographic deflection is actually produced (fig. 15).

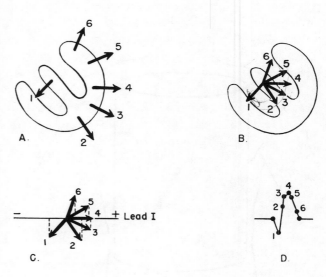

Fig. 15. (A) Diagram illustrating the frontal plane projection of the instantaneous QRS vectors. (B) The instantaneous QRS vectors drawn from a common origin. (C) Diagram illustrating the projection of the various instantaneous vectors on the Lead I axis. (D) The deflection produced by the instantaneous electrical forces illustrated in (C). It is seen that when the vector points toward the negative electrode, a downward deflection is written, and when a vector points toward the positive electrode, a positive deflection is written.

How to Determine the Direction of Electrical Forces in the Frontal Plane. With the lead axes and polarity of the hexaxial reference system in mind, it becomes a simple matter to determine the frontal plane direction of the P, QRS, ST, and T forces of the heart. This is done quickly and relatively accurately by simple inspection of the six extremity leads. The following discussion will be concerned with only the mean QRS force, but similar principles hold in calculating other mean and instantaneous vectors.

The direction of the mean QRS force is determined as follows: If the total QRS deflection on one lead is found to have as much area above the isoelectric line as below it, or is resultantly zero, the mean QRS must be perpendicular to that lead. From the QRS deflections in the other leads, it is a simple matter to determine on which side of the lead axis the arrow is drawn. Note that when mean vectors are being calculated, the total deflection is studied and its enclosed area, not its amplitude alone, is used to

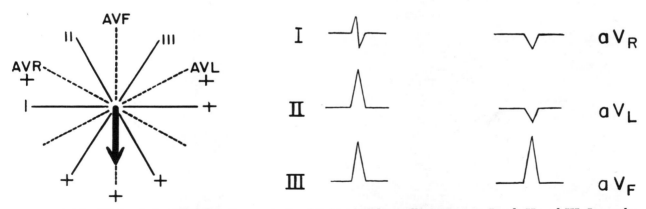

Fig. 16. The QRS complex is resultantly zero in Lead I, large and equally positive in Leads II and III. It can be represented by a mean vector directed downward and perpendicular to Lead I. Leads aV$_R$ and aV$_L$ are equally negative, and Lead aV$_F$ is large and positive for a mean vector with this direction.

23

determine the relative size of a deflection. In practice, it is perhaps easier to inspect the bipolar limb leads first and tentatively plot the vector direction and then check and correct it by inspecting the unipolar extremity leads. In fig. 16 the QRS is resultantly zero in Lead I and is, therefore, drawn perpendicular to Lead I. The deflections are equally positive in Leads II and III, and, therefore, the vector is drawn downward instead of upward. It can be seen that a mean vector with this direction has its largest projection on Lead aV$_F$ and will record the largest positive deflection in Lead aV$_F$. Its projection on Lead aV$_R$ and aV$_L$ is smaller, producing equal but negative deflections in aV$_R$ and aV$_L$.

If inspection of the three bipolar extremity leads reveals that the resultant QRS complex is conspicuously larger on one lead than on the other two leads, then the mean QRS vector will be relatively parallel to that lead. In fig. 17, the QRS complex is largest in Lead II; therefore, the mean QRS vector is parallel to Lead II, and

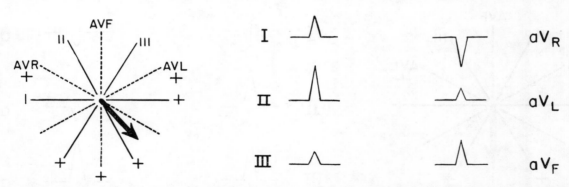

Fig. 17. The QRS complex is largest and positive on Lead II and less large but still positive on Leads I and III. The mean QRS vector would be tentatively drawn parallel with Lead II. Since the QRS complex is resultantly slightly positive in Lead aV$_L$, the mean QRS vector must be rotated slightly to the left.

is directed so that Leads I and II are positive. In this case, Lead aV$_L$ is in a critical position. If the vector is perfectly parallel to Lead II, Lead aV$_L$ should be resultantly zero. In this case, aV$_L$ is slightly positive and the vector must be adjusted so it will project a small positive quantity on the lead axis of aV$_L$.

By using the six extremity lead axes in such a manner, one can learn to locate the direction of a vector with an accuracy of about plus or minus 5°. The vector positions lying between those shown above can be determined by interpolation and constantly recalling that Lead I plus III equals Lead II and that aV$_R$ plus aV$_L$ plus aV$_F$ equals zero.

The direction of a vector gives enough clinical information and its size and magnitude need not be established in absolute terms. If the QRS complex contains a certain area and the T waves contain roughly half that area, then it is satisfactory to draw the mean QRS vector twice as long as the mean T vector, thereby indicating their relative magnitudes.

The Precordial Leads. The precordial leads can be used to determine the anterior or posterior deviation or a vector out of the frontal plane. The precordial electrode positions were apparently originally chosen because it was believed that "samples" of the right and left ventricular electrical forces could be recorded from such points. This is probably not a sound assumption, but to prevent confusion, the same electrode positions are retained and are as follows:

V-1. Fourth intercostal space just to the right of the sternum.

V-2. Fourth intercostal space just to the left of the sternum.

V-3. Midpoint on a line connecting V-2 and V-4.

V-4. Fifth intercostal space on the midclavicular line.

V-5. At the same level as V-4 on the anterior axillary line.

V-6. At the same level as V-4 on the midaxillary line.

For many years bipolar chest leads were used. This type of lead was accomplished by placing the lead wire of the positive pole of the galvanometer on the chest and the lead wire of the negative pole on a relatively remote extremity.

The evidence is now overwhelming in assuring the superiority of the Wilson unipolar precordial leads, the V leads, over the bipolar chest leads. When V leads are used, the exploring electrode is placed on the chest and is attached to the positive pole of the galvanometer while to the negative pole of the galvanometer is attached a central terminal made up of wire connections to the right arm, left arm, and left leg. This is, of course, the same network and connections used to record unaugmented unipolar extremity leads except for the fact that the exploring electrode is placed on the chest rather than the extremities.

It is not necessary to augment or increase the magnitude of the precordial leads since their electrode positions are so much nearer the source of electrical energy than are the extremity electrode positions.

The precordial electrode positions are shown on the diagram of the human chest in fig. **18A**. The small dot in the center of the chest indicates the approximate location of the origin of electrical force produced by the heart. The origin of electrical activity is satisfactorily considered to be roughly 2 to 3 centimeters below the level of the V-1 and V-2 precordial electrode positions in the center of the chest. In reality, the origin of the electrical force is probably not centrally located and varies from subject to subject but for simplicity is regarded to be at a centrally located fixed point.

When the chest is considered to be a cylinder, which is reasonable from an electrical point of

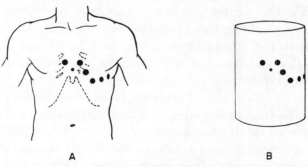

A   B

Fig. 18. (A) The electrode positions of the chest leads are illustrated. The small dot in the center of the chest indicates the approximate location of the origin of electrical forces of the heart (2 to 3 cm. below the level of V-1 and V-2 electrode positions). (B) The electrode positions diagrammed on a cylindrical replica of the chest.

view, the precordial electrode positions and the origin of electrical force can be indicated on the cylinder (fig. 18B). Certain shortcomings in assuming the chest to be a cylinder as shown in fig. 18B will be discussed later.

Certain aspects of the unipolar precordial leads deserve additional comment. The axes of these leads can be visualized by drawing a line from the exploring chest electrode through the origin of the electrical force to the opposite side of the chest. The direction of the six axes will vary from subject to subject, depending on chest contour and therefore do not have a mathematical relationship with each other as do the extremity lead axes. As with the extremity leads, when an electrical force is directed toward a V lead precordial electrode, it will produce a positive deflection on that lead and when an electrical force is directed away from such an electrode, it will produce a negative deflection on that lead. The axes of V-1 and V-2 are nearly perpendicular to the frontal plane and, therefore, an electrical force which is parallel with the frontal plane will hardly influence the V-1 and V-2 electrodes. The lead axis of V-6, being in the midaxillary line, is almost a frontal plane lead and will frequently resemble Lead I. The lead axes of V-3, V-4, and V-5 are influenced by frontal plane as well as anteroposteriorly directed forces.

In fig. 19 the spatial characteristics of the electrical field produced by a vector perpendicular to Lead III and parallel with the frontal plane is diagrammatically illustrated. When the electrical field is viewed spatially, the zone of zero potential becomes a plane dividing the chest or cylinder into negative and positive halves. It can be seen that the electrodes for Leads V-2, V-3, V-4, V-5, V-6 are recording from the positive zone of the electrical field and that the electrode for Lead V-1 is recording from the negative zone of the electrical field. The line on the surface where the zero potential plane intersects the surface of the chest, or cylinder, is called the transitional pathway for that vector. Transitional complexes are recorded by electrodes placed on the transitional pathway (fig. 19). The precordial lead with the largest deflection cannot be considered to be parallel with the electrical force since some of the chest elec-

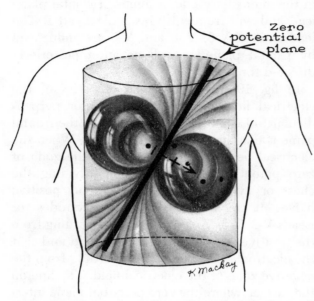

Zero potential plane

K. mackay

FIG. 19. Diagrammatic "spatial view" of an electrical field produced by a force perpendicular to Lead III. The zero potential plane extends to intersect the surface of the cylinder to produce the transitional pathway. In this case Lead V-1 records from the negative portion of the electrical field and Leads V-2, V-3, V-4, V-5, V-6 record from the positive portion of the electrical field. V lead electrodes placed on the transitional pathway record transitional complexes.

trodes are nearer the heart than others and will record larger deflections for this reason. On the other hand the precordial electrode which records the transitional complex can be considered to be on an axis perpendicular to the electrical force since it lies on the transitional pathway and the position of the pathway is determined by the direction of the force and not its magnitude (fig. 20).

After defining the direction of a vector in the frontal plane as described previously, the location of the transitional pathway will enable one to determine how far anteriorly or posteriorly the vector deviates from the frontal plane. When one considers only an instantaneous vector or "single electrical force," the transitional pathway is identified by finding the precordial V lead where the force is isoelectric at the time the force is generated. When a mean vector is considered, the transitional pathway is identified by finding the precordial lead where the total deflection is resultantly zero. A complex which is resultantly zero is often termed an equiphasic or transitional complex, that is, it encloses as much area above the line as below.

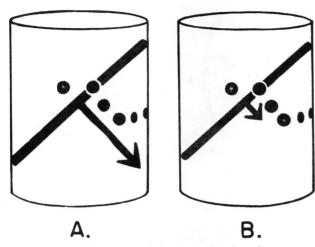

A.   B.

Fig. 20. The location of the transitional pathway produced by the large vector in (A) is the same as that produced by the small vector in (B).

To illustrate how the location of the transitional pathway combined with the frontal plane direction of a vector enables one to orientate the vector in space, it is instructive to allow a vector to retain the same frontal plane position but to rotate it anteriorly or posteriorly and identify the area of negativity, positivity, and the plane of zero potential. In fig. 21, a vector is shown drawn perpendicular to Lead aV$_F$ and rotated posteriorly and anteriorly. Note how the location of the transitional complex would identify the plane of zero potential which is perpendicular to the vector.

From fig. 21, it should be obvious that the direction of a vector determines the zone of relative positivity and relative negativity and the location of the transitional pathway. Stated in another way, identification of the transitional pathway by locating the transitional complex identifies the direction of the vector since it is perpendicular to the vector.

Using the precordial leads to determine the extent to which a vector is anteriorly or posteriorly directed has limitations. If the electrodes are not properly placed, one will end up with an incorrect notion of where the transitional pathway crosses the precordium. Furthermore, the electrode positions will vary from person to person depending on chest contour even though the positions have been properly located from an anatomic point of view. If the chest is broad, the electrode positions of V-2, V-3, and V-4 tend to be in the same horizontal line and if the chest

29

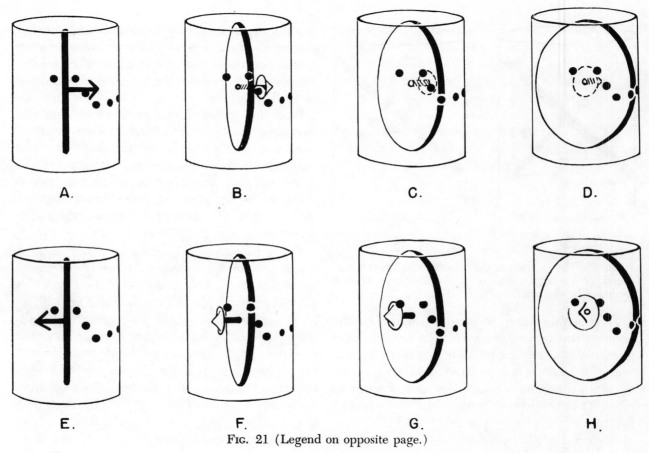

A.   B.   C.   D.

E.   F.   G.   H.

FIG. 21 (Legend on opposite page.)

is thin and long, these electrode positions tend to be more vertically placed one above the other (fig. 22). Hence, finding a transitional complex at position V-4 would actually be due to a more posteriorly directed vector in a broad-chested subject than in a thin-chested subject.

Only one size of cylinder will be utilized in the illustrations in the remainder of this book. This is done for the sake of simplicity and at the expense of accuracy since it is virtually impossible to draw an electrical cylinder for every chest. Because of this unknown quantity, precordial leads cannot define a vector position as accurately as extremity leads and the range of error is probably about 15°. In practice the gross variations in chest size and contour may often be inferred from body weight, height, and other clinical data. The accuracy of interpretation will always be enhanced by knowing these data.

At times, it may be found necessary to obtain additional chest leads, particularly over the right side of the chest in anteriorly directed vectors for it is fairly common to find all T waves upright in the usual precordial leads. In order to locate the transitional pathway in such a case, leads to the right of V-1 may be necessary. In

---

FIG. 21. (A) When the vector is directed to the left and is flush with the frontal plane, V-1 will record a negative deflection and V-2, V-3, V-4, V-5, and V-6 will record positive deflections. (B) When the vector is rotated 10° posteriorly, V-1 will record a negative deflection, V-2 will be resultantly zero, and V-3, V-4, V-5, and V-6 will record positive deflections. (C) When the vector is rotated 40° posteriorly, V-1, V-2, V-3 will record negative deflections, V-4 will be resultantly zero, and V-5 and V-6 will record positive deflections. (D) When the vector is rotated 70° to 80° posteriorly, V-1, V-2, V-3, V-4, and V-5 will record negative deflections, and V-6 will record a positive deflection. (E) When the vector is directed to the right and is flush with the frontal plane, V-1 will record a positive deflection, and V-2, V-3, V-4, V-5, and V-6 will record negative deflections. (F) When the vector is rotated 10° anteriorly, V-1 will record a positive deflection, V-2 will be resultantly zero, and V-3, V-4, V-5, and V-6 will record negative deflections. (G) When the vector is rotated 40° anteriorly, V-1, V-2, V-3 will record positive deflections, V-4 will be resultantly zero, and V-5 and V-6 will record negative deflections. (H) When the vector is rotated 70° to 80° anteriorly, V-1, V-2, V-3, V-4, and V-5 will record positive deflections, and V-6 will record a negative deflection.

31

this way one can determine how far anteriorly the vector is rotated.

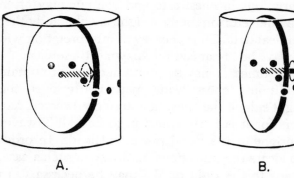

A. **B.**

Fig. 22. (A) A cylinder representing a large, broadchested, subject. (B) A cylinder representing a thin, long-chested, subject. The transitional pathway passes through electrode position V-4 in each instance but the vector is rotated more posteriorly in (A) than in (B).

Summary of the Procedure Used to Determine the Spatial Direction of Electrical Forces Illustrated as Vectors: *Step 1.* Determine the frontal plane direction of the mean QRS and T vectors by inspecting the bipolar limb leads and then alter their directions to satisfy the unipolar limb leads (fig. 23). This can be quickly accomplished by recalling that when an electrical force is relatively parallel with a given lead axis, it records its largest deflection on that lead and when an electrical force is relatively perpendicular to a given lead axis, it records its smallest deflection on that lead. The polarity of the leads must be kept in mind.

Step 2. Visualize the mean QRS vector within a cylinder. The frontal plane position as determined in Step 1 is retained and its origin is located in the center of the cylinder. The mean T vector is then visualized in a like manner.

Step 3. Inspect the unipolar precordial leads and identify the transitional QRS and T complexes. (A transitional complex is defined as a deflection which is equally negative and positive or resultantly zero.)

Step 4. Consider the QRS vector tilted posteriorly or anteriorly, as the case may be, to a point where the zero potential plane of the QRS vector will pass through the electrode position which records the transitional complex. The mean T vector is then treated similarly.

The QRS Loop. It is useful, though not necessary, for one to be able to illustrate the spatial instantaneous vectors producing the QRS deflections by drawing the spatial QRS loop. The spatial QRS loop enables one to visualize the change in magnitude and direction of vectors from instant to instant in a single QRS cycle. A simple way to draw the spatial QRS loop is illustrated and described in fig. 24.

The Initial and Terminal Mean .04 Vectors. While it is seldom necessary for one to construct the details of the spatial QRS loop, it is frequently necessary for one to calculate a mean vector for the forces generated during the initial and terminal .04 second of the QRS loop. Ac-

cordingly, the method for determining the direction of a mean vector representing the forces generated during the initial and terminal .04 second for the QRS loop is described and illustrated in fig. 25.

In this chapter the method for determining the spatial direction of electrical forces generated by the heart has been described. In the following chapters it will be shown how an electrocardiogram can be interpreted by studying the direction of the various electrical forces and their relationship to each other.

FIG. 23. An electrocardiogram with the QRS and T deflections represented by mean spatial vectors. (A) The frontal plane projection of the mean spatial QRS and T vectors. The resultant QRS deflection is approximately equal in Leads II and III and is slightly negative in Lead I. The largest deflection in the unipolar extremity leads is in Lead aV_F and the deflection is positive. These QRS characteristics can be represented by a mean QRS vector directed relatively parallel to Lead aV_F but rotated to the right just enough for a small negative quantity to be projected on Lead I. The T wave is largest and positive in Lead I and smallest in Lead III. When a long strip of Lead III is studied, the T wave is seen to vary with respiration but is most often slightly negative. These T wave characteristics can be represented by a mean vector directed just to the left of a perpendicular to Lead III. The largest negative deflection will therefore be recorded in Lead aV_R. (B) The mean spatial QRS vector oriented in the cylindrical replica of the chest. The QRS vector must be rotated 20° posteriorly because the transitional pathway passes between electrode positions V-3 and V-4. (C) The mean spatial T vector oriented in the cylindrical replica of the chest. The mean T vector must be rotated 50° posteriorly because the transitional pathway passes between electrode positions V-4 and V-5. (D) Final summary figure illustrating the mean spatial QRS and T vectors. The rim of the arrow tip is oriented spatially so that it parallels the transitional pathway of that particular vector and produces a three-dimensional effect.

34

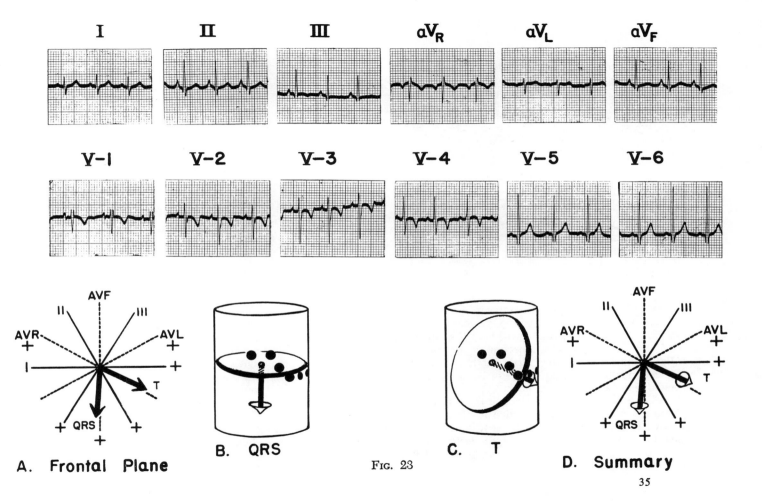

I II III aVR aVL aVF

V-1 V-2 V-3 V-4 V-5 V-6

A. Frontal Plane

B. QRS

C. T

D. Summary

Fig. 23

35

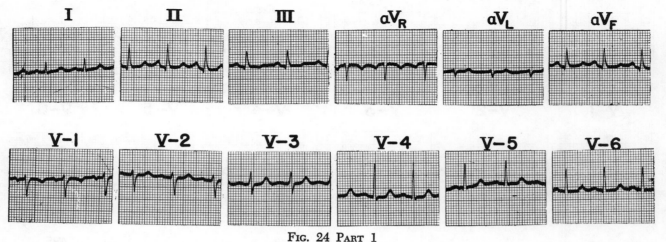

FIG. 24 PART 1

FIG. 24. Part I. A normal electrocardiogram.

Part II. How to construct the QRS loop. In this illustration the tracing shown in Part I is used as an example.

(A) The frontal plane projection of the mean spatial QRS vector is established first. In this case the QRS deflection is largest and positive in Lead II and slightly negative in Lead aV$_L$. The mean QRS vector will therefore be directed just to the right of the positive limb of Lead II. A simple, rough outline of the QRS loop is drawn to satisfy the deflection recorded from the lead axis located nearest to the mean QRS vector. In this case a simple loop is drawn to satisfy the Lead II deflection.

Accordingly, a small initial portion of the loop (less than .02 second) must project a small negative quantity on Lead II and the remaining portion (.06 second) must project large positive quantities on Lead II.

(B) The simple QRS loop constructed in (A) is next altered to satisfy the three bipolar extremity leads. In this case Lead III must have a small initial negative deflection and the remaining portion of the QRS deflection must be positive. The simple outline drawn in (A) is satisfactory in regard to Lead III. The loop must be altered so that an initial small negative deflection can be recorded in Lead I. The initial negative deflection is

(Legend continued on page 38.)

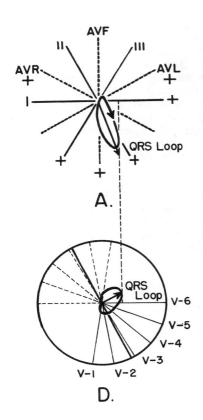

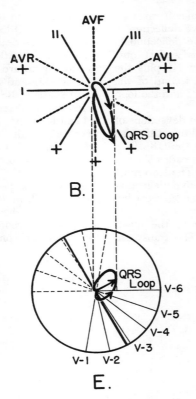

A. B. C.

D. E. F.

Transverse Plane D, E, and F

FIG. 24. PART 2

so small in Lead I that it is hardly visible. It must be present, however, since the initial negative deflection in Lead II is larger than the initial negative deflection in Lead III and the deflection magnitude of Lead II must equal the deflection magnitude of Lead III plus the magnitude of Lead I. The terminal .02 second of the QRS complex is slightly negative in Lead I and the loop must be altered so that this can occur.

(C) The loop constructed to satisfy the deflections of the bipolar extremity leads is now altered to satisfy also the unipolar extremity leads. In this case the QRS loop shown in (B) is satisfactory in regard to Leads aV_R and aV_F but is not satisfactory for Lead aV_L. The loop must be altered so that an initial small positive deflection followed by a larger negative deflection can be recorded in Lead aV_L.

(D) The transverse plane projection of the mean spatial QRS vector is established next. The transverse plane can be visualized by facing the subject and inspecting the QRS loop from above. Note in (A) the dotted line is drawn perpendicular to Lead I through the arrow tip of the mean QRS vector. This line is continued downward in the drawing to intersect the V-6 axis of (D) and therefore indicates how much of the mean spatial QRS vector can be seen from above. The precordial lead recording the transitional QRS complex is identified next. The mean QRS vector is directed perpendicular to the lead axis which records the transitional QRS complex. In this case, the deflection recorded at electrode position V-3 is almost transitional but is resultantly slightly positive. Accordingly, the lead axis from which a perfect transitional complex would be recorded will be located approximately as indicated by the heavy line shown in (D), (E), and (F). (Note that the complex recorded at V-2 is resultantly more negative than the complex recorded at V-3 is resultantly positive. Therefore an electrode placed nearer V-3 than V-2 would record a transitional complex.) The mean QRS vector is directed perpendicular to the heavy lead axis line and extends to intersect the dotted line which represents the extent to which the vector can be seen from above. A simple outline of the QRS loop is then drawn to encompass the mean QRS vector and should roughly satisfy the lead recording the precordial transitional QRS complex.

(E) The transverse QRS loop constructed in (D) is now altered to satisfy the deflections recorded at electrode positions V-1, V-2, and V-3. Two dotted lines are shown drawn perpendicular to Lead I in (B) and continued downward to intersect the axis of Lead V-6 in (E). The transverse QRS loop must lie within the two dotted lines since it cannot extend a greater distance to the right or left. In this case the deflection in Lead V-1 has a small initial positive deflection and a larger negative deflection. Accordingly, the initial portion of the loop must be directed toward the V-1 electrode while the remaining portion of the loop must be negative to Lead V-1. The same situation exists regarding the deflection recorded in V-2. The loop must be drawn so that Lead V-3 can record a complex which is nearly transitional but resultantly slightly positive.

(F) The transverse QRS loop constructed in (E) is next altered to satisfy the deflections recorded at electrode positions V-4, V-5, and V-6. In this case the loop must be changed so that Lead V-4 can record a small initial negative deflection of .01 second duration followed by a large positive deflection of .04 second duration which is followed by a small terminal negative deflection of .03 second duration. Since Lead V-5 records barely visible and brief initial and terminal negative deflections, the loop must be altered so that such can occur. The QRS duration in V-6 appears narrow because the initial and terminal instantaneous forces are approximately perpendicular to the lead axis of V-6.

FIG. 25. How to determine the direction of the mean spatial initial and terminal .04 vectors. The mean spatial initial .04 vector represents the resultant of all forces generated during the initial .04 second of the QRS cycle. This vector becomes abnormally directed after myocardial infarction and points away from the area of dead muscle. The mean spatial terminal .04 vector represents the resultant of all forces generated during the terminal .04 second of the QRS cycle. The direction of this vector aids one in determining the type of bundle branch block in cases where the QRS duration is prolonged beyond .12 second.

(A) The frontal plane projection of the mean QRS, initial .04, and terminal .04 vectors. The QRS deflection is large and positive in Lead I and resultantly slightly positive in Lead aV$_F$. The mean QRS vector will therefore be directed to the left and will be relatively parallel with Lead I but located so that a small positive quantity will be projected on Lead aV$_F$. The basic principles used to determine the direction of the mean QRS vector are used in determining the directions of the mean initial and terminal .04 vectors. Because of the difficulty the beginner encounters in determining the directions of the initial and terminal .04 vectors, each lead will be studied separately, thereby gradually narrowing the area where the .04 vector under study may lie. In this case the initial .04 second of the QRS cycle is resultantly positive in Lead I. Therefore the initial .04 vector must be directed somewhere in the semicircle located to the left of the axis of Lead aV$_F$. The initial .04 second of the QRS cycle is resultantly positive in Lead II and therefore the initial .04 vector must lie somewhere between the positive limb of Lead aV$_L$ and the positive limb of Lead aV$_F$. (The latter line of limitation having been established by studying Lead I.) The initial .04 second of the QRS cycle is resultantly slightly negative in Lead III and therefore the initial .04 vector must lie between the negative limb of aV$_R$ and the positive limb of Lead aV$_L$. (The latter line of limitation having been established by studying Lead II.) This area, limited on the one side by the positive limb of Lead aV$_L$ and on the other side by the negative limb of Lead aV$_R$, will satisfy the findings in Lead aV$_L$ and aV$_R$ since a vector located in this area will record an initial resultantly negative deflection in Lead aV$_R$ and a resultantly positive deflection in Lead aV$_L$. The initial .04 second of the QRS cycle is resultantly positive in Lead aV$_F$ thereby establishing the fact that the mean initial .04 vector must be directed between the positive limb of Lead I and the negative limb of Lead aV$_R$. (The latter line of limitation having been established by studying Lead III.) Since the initial .04 second of the QRS cycle is resultantly only slightly negative in Lead III, the mean QRS vector is nearly perpendicular to Lead III. The direction of the mean terminal .04 vector is determined in the same manner as that of the mean initial .04 vector. Briefly, the terminal .04 second of the QRS cycle is negative in Leads II and aV$_R$. Accordingly, the

(Legend continued on page 42.)

40

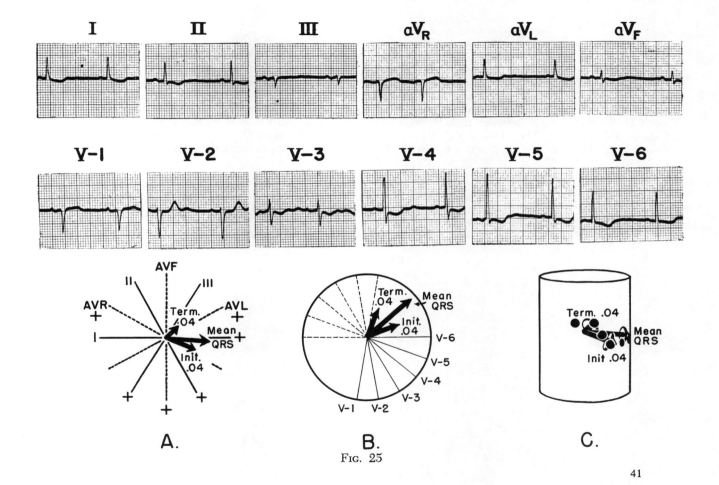

I   II   III   aV_R   aV_L   aV_F

V-1   V-2   V-3   V-4   V-5   V-6

A.   B.   C.

Fig. 25

mean terminal .04 vector must lie between the positive limb of Lead aV_L and the negative limb of Lead III.

(B) The transverse plane projection of the mean QRS, initial, and terminal .04 vectors. The mean QRS vector is directed moderately posteriorly (approximately 40° to 45°) because the transitional pathway for the mean QRS vector passes between the electrode positions of V-3 and V-4. The mean initial .04 vector is directed slightly posteriorly (approximately 15° to 20°) because the initial .04 second of the QRS cycle is resultantly negative in V-1 and V-2 and resultantly positive in Leads V-3, V-4, V-5, and V-6. The mean terminal .04 vector is directed markedly posteriorly (approximately 70° to 80°) because the terminal .04 second of the QRS cycle is resultantly negative in Leads V-1, V-2, V-3, V-4, and V-5, and resultantly positive in Lead V-6.

(C) The mean QRS, initial, and terminal .04 vectors oriented in the cylindrical replica of the chest.

CHAPTER TWO

The Normal Ventricular Electrocardiogram

In the first chapter the method was described for determining the spatial direction of the underlying electrical forces which produce the electrocardiographic deflection. In the following chapters it will be shown how the electrocardiogram can be interpreted by studying these spatial electrical forces and their relationship to each other. The obvious first step in such a presentation is to describe the normal range of such forces. The abnormal electrocardiogram can then be established as a deviation from the normal.

The portion of the electrocardiogram produced by the ventricular musculature, including the QRS complex, the T wave, and ST segment displacement, can be represented by spatial vectors and utilized to study the electrocardiogram. The vector method of electrocardiography does not aid in the recognition of arrhythmias, and such cardiac disorders are not included in this discussion.

The QRS Vector. In general the mean spatial QRS vector is directed toward the area of greatest ventricular muscle mass, the right ventricle being predominant in the newborn and the left ventricle being predominant in the adult. In addition the direction of the mean spatial QRS vector is altered by the cardiac rotation associated with growth, and varies with body build. The duration of the QRS complex varies with age and should not exceed .1 second in the normal adult. The QRS loop should be studied. It usually suffices to study the initial and terminal forces composing the QRS loop and it is not necessary, in most instances, to construct the details of the entire loop.

The electrical "position" of the heart is identified by the location of the mean spatial QRS vector and the detailed patterns for the various positions need not be memorized.

The T Vector. The T wave, representing repolarization, is written during ventricular systole and appears to be influenced by the pressure gradient across the ventricular muscle. This pressure gradient varies with the thickness of the ventricular muscle and the degree of intraventricular pressure. In the normal adult the muscle thickness and intraventricular pressure relationship is such that the T vector is directed relatively parallel with the mean QRS vector; however, in the newborn and child the pressure gradient across the ventricular muscle is quite different from that in the adult and the mean T vector is directed away from the right ventricle.

The QRS-T Angle. The spatial QRS-T angle, representing the relationship between the forces of depolarization and the forces of repolarization, varies with age. This variation will be emphasized in the discussion of the electrocardiograms that will follow. The QRS-T angle is a very useful tool. For example, in the average adult the spatial QRS-T angle is seldom wider than 60°. When angles of 100° or 180° are found, this identifies an abnormal T vector for that particular QRS vector. The abnormal T vectors associated with a wide QRS-T angle will be discussed later.

The T vector should have a certain spatial position relative to the QRS vector even when the QRS-T angle is normal. Stated another way, a T vector may be abnormal when the QRS-T angle is normal if it does not have the proper and expected position for that particular QRS vector.

The ST Vector. Frequently a rather large ST vector is encountered in a normal subject and the spatial characteristics of such a vector should be defined. The normal mean spatial ST vector is usually directed relatively parallel with the mean spatial T vector and represents early forces of repolarization occurring during the ST interval. Such an ST vector is usually associated with a large T vector. The normal ST vector can be differentiated from the ST vector of pericarditis, subendocardial ischemia, and potassium effect by its stability and lack of associated abnormalities on follow-up tracings.

The electrocardiograms that follow will serve as a background to enlarge on the foregoing statements.

The Normal Newborn. The electrical forces producing the neonatal electrocardiogram vary greatly from subject to subject. The mean QRS spatial vector is directed to the right and can be found within the wide limits shown in fig. 26A. The QRS vector is usually flush with the frontal plane or is tilted moderately anteriorly. Frequently the QRS complexes are diaphasic in the

extremity and precordial leads. Such deflections are the result of a rotund QRS loop. In other words, the initial forces composing the QRS loop are directed in one direction, whereas the terminal forces may be directed in an opposite direction. The transitional pathway on the chest is much broader than in the adult and difficulty may be encountered in identifying a perfect transitional complex since many of the complexes appear equiphasic.

The mean spatial T vector is usually directed to the left and can be found anywhere within the wide limits shown in fig. 26B. The T vector is usually rotated moderately posteriorly but on rare occasions has been found to be directed anteriorly and may vary in direction from hour to hour during the early period of life.

In the normal newborn's electrocardiogram the spatial QRS-T angle varies between 90° and 160° (fig. 27).

Two Years of Age. (See fig. 28.) By the age of two the QRS vector has rotated toward the left and comes to lie very nearly parallel with the positive portion of Lead II. In addition it becomes tilted slightly posteriorly. The T vector

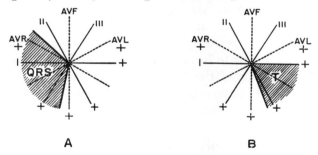

A   B

Fig. 26. (A) The mean QRS vector of the newborn can be found within the wide limits of the shaded area shown above. (B) The mean T vector of the newborn can be found within the wide limits of the shaded area shown above.

rotates to become fairly parallel with the QRS vector in the frontal plane but may retain a moderately posterior position. The spatial QRS-T angle is usually less than 45° but may be as much as 90° when the T vector retains a posterior position.

Childhood and Adolescence. (See figs. 29, 30, 31.) During this period the mean QRS and T vectors may retain their frontal plane positions which is fairly parallel or even to the left of the positive limb of Lead II. The QRS vector begins to rotate more posteriorly and the T vector begins to rotate more anteriorly but may retain a posterior position.

The Young Adult. (See fig. 32.) During the teen-age period it is not uncommon to see the mean QRS vector rotated to the right and become more vertical than it was during childhood. This may be due to cardiac rotation secondary to a change in body build or to certain as yet unexplained factors. The posterior direction of the QRS which is established in early life persists throughout the remaining age groups. The QRS-T angle is usually about 45°, but again a normal posteriorly directed T vector may enlarge the

angle. The moderately posteriorly directed T vector, so common in childhood, may persist during the teen-age period, and on rare occasions may be seen during the third decade of life. This has been termed retention of the juvenile pattern. In the older age group one must differentiate the normal persistence of a juvenile T vector from an abnormality by correlating the electrocardiogram with the clinical data.

The Normal Adult. (See figs. 33, 34, 35, 36.) In general, one can state that the frontal plane position of the mean spatial QRS vector will be directed either vertically, horizontally to the left, or toward an intermediate zone. In the normal subject the direction of the mean QRS vector seems to be nearly parallel with the anatomical axis of the heart. Thin, tall individuals frequently have vertically directed QRS vectors, and obese individuals with high diaphragms frequently have horizontally directed QRS vectors. The normal adult QRS vector, regardless of its frontal plane position, is always directed slightly posteriorly, the transitional complex in the precordial leads being usually seen at electrode position V-3 or V-4.

The QRS loop of the usual adult is more elongated than that of the newborn. The mean of electrical forces generated during the first .04 second of the QRS cycle, when represented as a vector, has a fairly definite relationship with the mean spatial QRS vector. This force is usually within 60° of the mean spatial QRS vector. The .04 vector should be directed to the left of the vertically placed QRS vector, to the right of the markedly horizontal QRS vector, and can lie on either side of the QRS vector in the intermediate position. The normal .04 vector is usually directed a few degrees anteriorly or may be flush with the frontal plane. Occasionally it may be rotated a few degrees posteriorly and produce deflections with absent R waves in Leads V-1 and V-2 but is never rotated to the degree that it is posterior to the mean QRS vector.

The mean T vector is usually directed to the left and may be flush with the frontal plane or tilted slightly posteriorly or anteriorly. The mean T vector should lie to the left of the vertically placed mean QRS vector, to the right of the markedly horizontal QRS vector, and can lie on either side of the QRS vector in the intermediate position. The normal T vector should be directed anterior to the mean QRS vector in almost all instances.

As stated previously, a measurable ST vector is frequently present in the normal subject, representing early repolarization, and is usually directed relatively parallel with the mean spatial T vector.

FIG. 27. The electrocardiogram of a normal two-day-old infant.

(A) The frontal plane projection of the mean spatial QRS, ST, and T vectors. The QRS complex is largest and negative in Lead I and resultantly slightly negative in Lead aV_F. QRS complexes of this nature can be represented by a mean vector directed relatively parallel with the Lead I axis. The mean QRS vector must be directed about 10° above the Lead I axis since it projects a small negative quantity on to the Lead aV_F axis. The resultant negativity of the QRS in Leads I and II indicate that the vector points to the right rather than to the left. The T wave is smallest in Lead III, upright in Leads II and III, and deeply inverted in Lead aV_R. Accordingly, the mean T vector is perpendicular to Lead III and is directed downward and to the left. The ST deviation appears largest and positive in Lead II and therefore the ST vector is parallel with Lead II.

(B) The mean spatial QRS vector oriented in the cylindrical replica of the chest. The QRS must be rotated 40° anteriorly so that the transitional pathway will pass between electrode positions V-3 and V-4. Note the diaphasic precordial complexes.

(C) The mean spatial T vector oriented in the cylindrical replica of the chest. The T vector must be rotated 20° posteriorly so that the transitional pathway will pass through electrode position V-3.

(D) The mean spatial ST vector oriented in the cylindrical replica of the chest. The ST vector must be rotated 30° posteriorly so that the transitional pathway will pass between electrode positions V-3 and V-4. (The ST segment is definitely negative in V-1, V-2, and V-3 and, when studied in a long strip of electrocardiogram, is very slightly positive in V-4, V-5, and V-6. The ST positivity is slight in V-4, V-5, and V-6 because these leads record near the transitional pathway and are recording from a greater distance than electrodes placed at V-1, V-2, and V-3.)

(E) Final summary figure illustrating a spatial QRS-T angle of 150°. The mean ST vector is nearly parallel with the mean T vector.

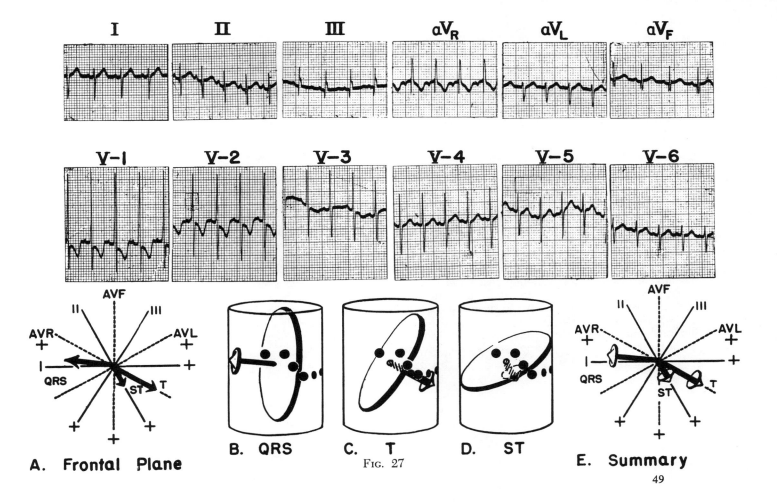

I II III aV_R aV_L aV_F

V-1 V-2 V-3 V-4 V-5 V-6

A. Frontal Plane

B. QRS   C. T   D. ST

E. Summary

Fig. 27

49

FIG. 28. The electrocardiogram of a normal child, age two.

(A) The frontal plane projection of the mean QRS and T vectors. The QRS complex is largest and positive on Lead II and slightly positive on Lead III and aV_L. QRS complexes of this nature can be represented by a mean vector directed just to the left of the positive limb of Lead II. The T wave is largest in Lead II, large and negative in Lead aV_R, and slightly positive in Lead III. Such T waves can be represented by a mean vector directed just to the right of a perpendicular to Lead III.

(B) The mean spatial QRS vector oriented in a cylindrical replica of the chest. Note that the QRS complex in V-1 varies with the respiratory cycle and that some of the complexes are transitional while others are negative. The transitional pathway is, therefore, slightly different with each phase of respiration. Since V-3, V-4, V-5, and V-6 are definitely positive, it is reasonable to place the transitional pathway so that the mean QRS is flush with the frontal plane. A vector so located would represent an average vector position for all phases of respiration.

(C) The mean spatial T vector oriented in a cylindrical replica of the chest. The T vector is rotated 20° posteriorly because the transitional pathway passes through electrode position V-3.

(D) Final summary figure illustrating a spatial QRS-T angle of 20°.

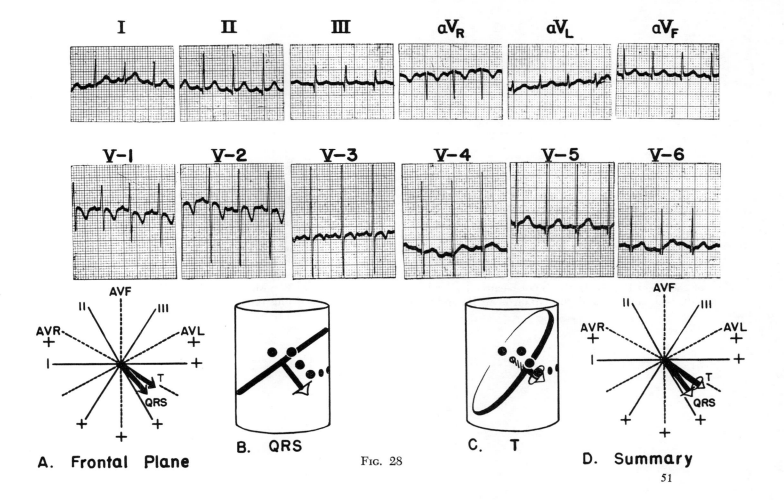

I II III aV$_R$ aV$_L$ aV$_F$

V-1 V-2 V-3 V-4 V-5 V-6

A. Frontal Plane   B. QRS   Fig. 28   C. T   D. Summary

51

FIG. 29. The electrocardiogram of a normal child, age three and one-half, illustrating the posteriorly directed T vector. (A) The frontal plane projection of the mean QRS and T vectors. The QRS complex is largest and positive on Lead II and slightly positive on Lead aV_L. QRS complexes of this nature can be represented by a mean vector directed just to the left of the positive limb of the Lead II axis. In the bipolar extremity leads the T wave is smallest and positive on Lead III and in the unipolar extremity leads the T wave is largest and negative in Lead aV_R. Under these circumstances the mean T vector will be directed just to the right of the negative limb of Lead axis aV_R. (B), (C) The mean spatial QRS and T vector oriented in cylindrical replicas of the chest. Both the QRS and T vectors are rotated approximately 30° posteriorly because their transitional pathways pass between electrode positions V-3 and V-4. (D) Final summary figure illustrating a spatial QRS-T angle of 20°.

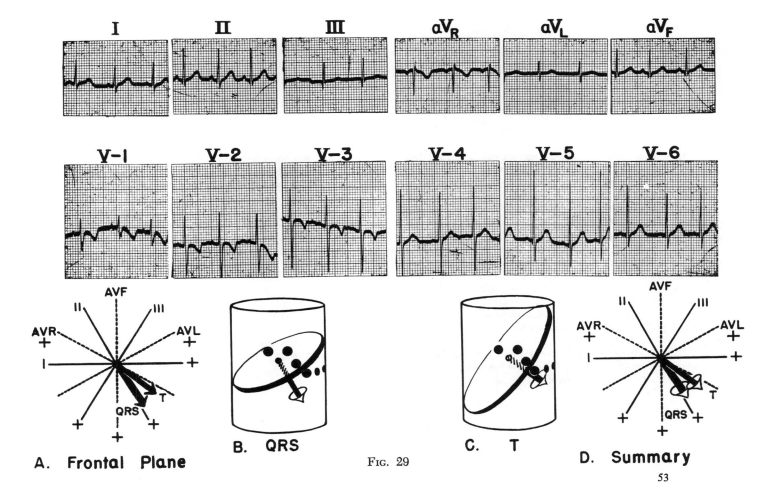

I II III aV_R aV_L aV_F

V-1 V-2 V-3 V-4 V-5 V-6

A. Frontal Plane

B. QRS

C. T

D. Summary

Fig. 29

Fig. 30. The electrocardiogram of a normal child, age six.

(A) The frontal plane projection of the mean QRS and T vectors. The QRS complex is smallest but positive in Lead III in the bipolar extremity leads but is largest and negative in Lead aV_R in the unipolar extremity leads. QRS complexes of this nature can be represented by a mean vector directed just to the right of a perpendicular to the Lead III axis. The T wave is largest and positive on Lead II but slightly positive on Lead aV_L. T waves of this nature can be represented by a mean vector directed just to the left of the Lead II axis.

(B) The mean spatial QRS vector oriented in the cylindrical replica of the chest. The QRS vector must be rotated approximately 15° posteriorly because the transitional pathway passes between the electrode positions V-2 and V-3.

(C) The mean spatial T vector oriented in the cylindrical replica of the chest. The T vector must be rotated approximately 10° posteriorly because the transitional pathway passes between the electrode positions V-2 and V-3.

(D) Final summary figure illustrating a spatial QRS-T angle of 5°. Note the multiphasic T waves in Lead V-2. These peculiar waves are produced because electrode position V-2 is recording very near the transitional pathway for the T wave. Under such circumstances some of the instantaneous T vectors project positive quantities in that lead while other instantaneous T vectors, located only a few degrees away, project negative quantities. In this case the early instantaneous T vectors are directed more posteriorly than the terminal instantaneous T vectors, producing a negative deflection during the early part of the T wave and a positive deflection during the last part of the T wave. The multiphasic contour is not seen in the other precordial T waves because all the instantaneous T vectors project either positive quantities or negative quantities on the other precordial lead axes.

54

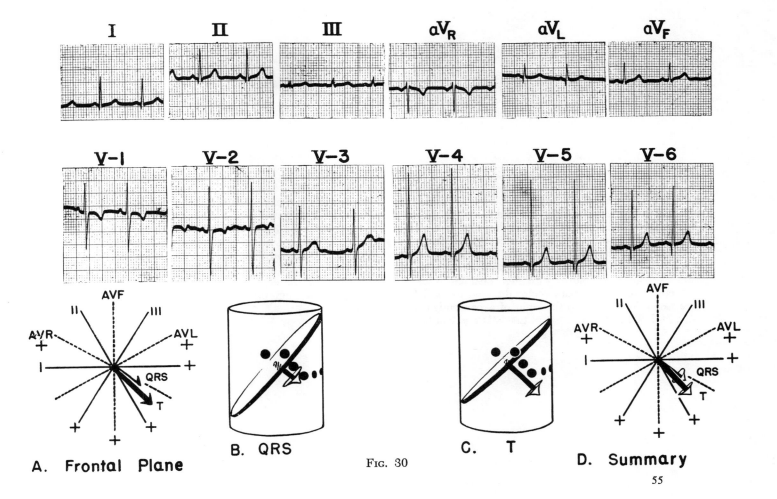

I II III aV_R aV_L aV_F

V-1 V-2 V-3 V-4 V-5 V-6

A. Frontal Plane

B. QRS

Fig. 30

C. T

D. Summary

55

Fɪɢ. 31. The electrocardiogram of a normal child, age 12, illustrating a posteriorly directed T vector. (Such a T vector position may occasionally be seen in a normal adult.) (A) The frontal plane projection of the mean QRS and T vectors. Note that the QRS is largest and positive on Lead II but slightly positive on Lead III and aV$_L$. QRS complexes with such characteristics can be represented by a mean vector directed to the left of the Lead II axis and to the right of a perpendicular to Lead III. The T wave is flat in Lead III and can be rep-resented by a mean vector directed perpendicular to Lead III. It is drawn to the left because the T wave is upright in Leads I and II. (B), (C) The mean spatial QRS and T vectors oriented in cylindrical replicas of the chest. The QRS and T vector must be rotated about 35° posteriorly so that the transitional pathway for both will pass between the electrode positions V-3 and V-4. (D) Final summary figure illustrating a spatial QRS-T angle of 15°.

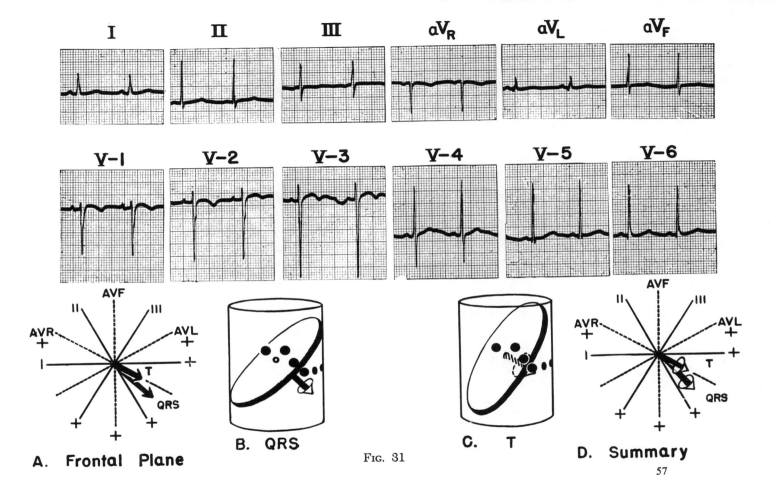

| I | II | III | aV_R | aV_L | aV_F |

| V-1 | V-2 | V-3 | V-4 | V-5 | V-6 |

A. Frontal Plane

B. QRS

Fig. 31

C. T

D. Summary

57

FIG. 32. The electrocardiogram of a normal subject, age 18. (A) The frontal plane projection of the mean QRS and T vectors. The QRS complex is largest on Lead II but slightly positive on Lead aV$_L$. These findings enable one to draw quickly the mean QRS vector just to the left of the Lead II axis. The T wave is smallest but slightly negative on Lead III and positive on Lead aV$_F$. These findings enable one to draw quickly the mean T vector to the left of a line perpendicular to Lead III. (B) The mean spatial QRS vector oriented in the cylindrical replica of the chest. The QRS vector is rotated approximately 15° posteriorly because the transitional pathway passes between the V-2 and V-3 electrode positions. (C) The mean spatial T vector oriented in cylindrical replica of the chest. The T vector is flush with the frontal plane because the transitional pathway for the T wave passes between the V-1 and V-2 electrode position. (D) Final summary figure illustrating a spatial QRS-T angle of 25°.

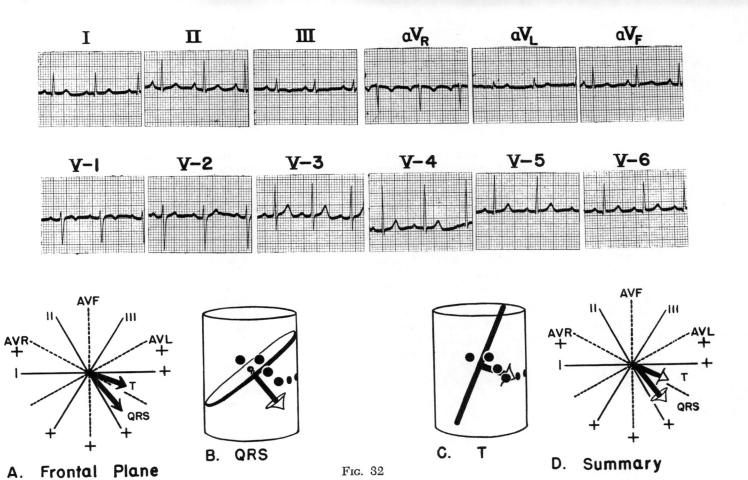

I II III aV_R aV_L aV_F

V-1 V-2 V-3 V-4 V-5 V-6

A. Frontal Plane

B. QRS

Fig. 32

C. T

D. Summary

Fig. 33. The electrocardiogram of a normal adult, age 40, illustrating a mean QRS vector in the intermediate position.

(A) The frontal plane projection of the mean spatial QRS and T vectors. The QRS complex is resultantly largest on Lead II and slightly positive on Lead aV_L, requiring that the mean QRS vector be drawn just to the left of the Lead II axis. A QRS vector so directed is said to be in an intermediate zone. The T wave is largest in Lead II and slightly positive in Lead aV_L. The T wave, represented as a vector, is located just to the left of the Lead II axis.

(B) The mean spatial QRS vector oriented in the cylindrical replica of the chest. The mean QRS vector is rotated approximately 30° posteriorly because the transitional pathway passes between electrode positions V-3 and V-4.

(C) The mean spatial T vector oriented in the cylindrical replica of the chest. The mean T vector is rotated at least 15° anteriorly because the V-1 electrode position records from the positive portion of the electrical field. When all the precordial T waves are upright it may be necessary to obtain leads to the right of the usual precordial lead positions in order to localize a vector position precisely. Since the T wave in Lead V-1 is smaller than the T wave in Lead V-6, one can assume that Lead V-1 was recording nearer the transitional pathway of the mean T vector than was Lead V-6. Accordingly, it is likely that the mean T vector is only slightly anteriorly directed.

(D) Final summary figure illustrating a spatial QRS-T angle of 45°.

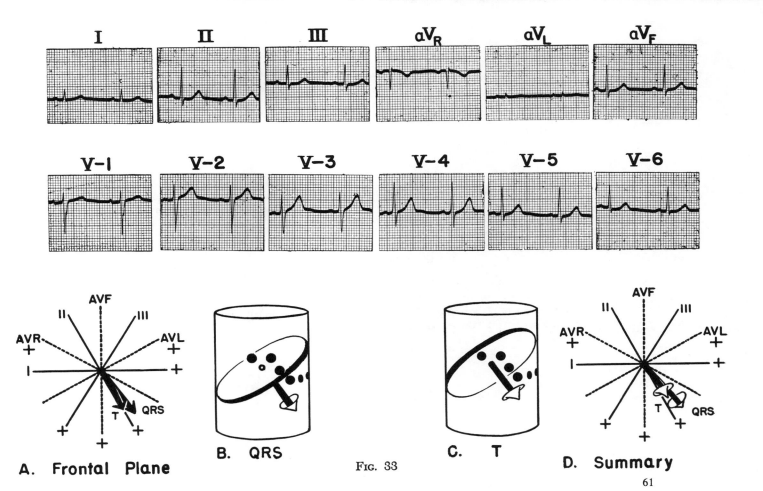

| I | II | III | aV$_R$ | aV$_L$ | aV$_F$ |

| V-1 | V-2 | V-3 | V-4 | V-5 | V-6 |

A. Frontal Plane   B. QRS   Fig. 33   C. T   D. Summary

61

FIG. 34. The electrocardiogram of a normal adult, age 51, illustrating a mean QRS vector in the horizontal position.

(A) The frontal plane projection of the mean spatial QRS and T vectors. The QRS is largest in Lead I and slightly negative in Lead aV_F. These findings in the extremity leads enable one to quickly place the mean QRS vector slightly to the left of the Lead I axis. Note that the QRS vector is pointing relatively far to the left. The T wave is largest in Lead I, slightly negative on Lead III, and slightly positive on Lead aV_F. These T wave characteristics illustrated as a vector are shown.

(B) The mean spatial QRS vector oriented in the cylindrical replica of the chest. The mean QRS vector is rotated approximately 20° posteriorly because the transitional pathway passes between electrode positions V-2 and V-3.

(C) The mean spatial T vector oriented in the cylindrical replica of the chest. The mean T vector is rotated approximately 5° anteriorly because its transitional pathway passes between electrode positions V-1 and V-2.

(D) Final summary figure illustrating a spatial QRS-T angle of 25°.

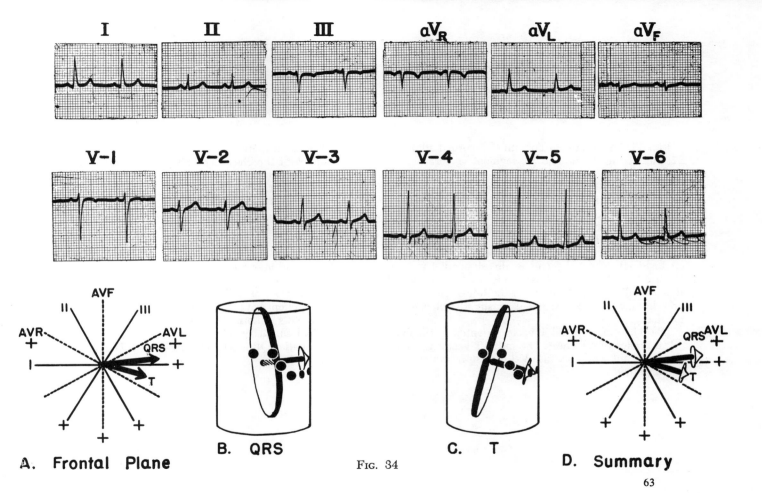

I   II   III   aV_R   aV_L   aV_F

V-1   V-2   V-3   V-4   V-5   V-6

A. Frontal Plane

B. QRS

Fig. 34

C. T

D. Summary

FIG. 35. The electrocardiogram of a normal adult, age 27, illustrating the normal ST segment vector.

(A) The frontal plane projection of the mean spatial QRS, ST, and T vectors. The mean QRS vector is almost parallel with Lead I since it is resultantly largest in Lead I. The QRS is slightly negative in Lead aV_F and therefore the QRS vector must be rotated slightly to the left of the positive limb of Lead I. The mean T vector is perpendicular to Lead III because the T wave is flat on Lead III. The ST vector is almost parallel to Lead II since the ST segment deviation is greatest on Lead II. It is actually located slightly to the left of such a position because the ST segment is slightly elevated in Lead aV_L.

(B) The mean spatial T vector oriented in the cylindrical replica of the chest. The mean T vector is rotated about 10° anteriorly because V-1 records from the transitional pathway.

(C) The mean spatial ST vector oriented in the cylindrical replica of the chest. The ST vector is directed a few more degrees anteriorly than the T vector since it is more positive at V-1.

(D) The mean spatial ST and T vectors superimposed. The mean spatial ST vector is nearly parallel with the mean spatial T vector. If a lead were recorded from the right, lower, anterior part of the chest, a resultantly negative QRS complex associated with an elevated ST segment and inverted T wave would be found. This finding would resemble the pattern of myocardial infarction. However, as will be seen, the vectors of myocardial infarction have altogether different directions from the vectors of normal persons.

(E) Final summary figure showing relationships of the mean spatial QRS, ST, and T vectors. The spatial QRS-T angle is 40°.

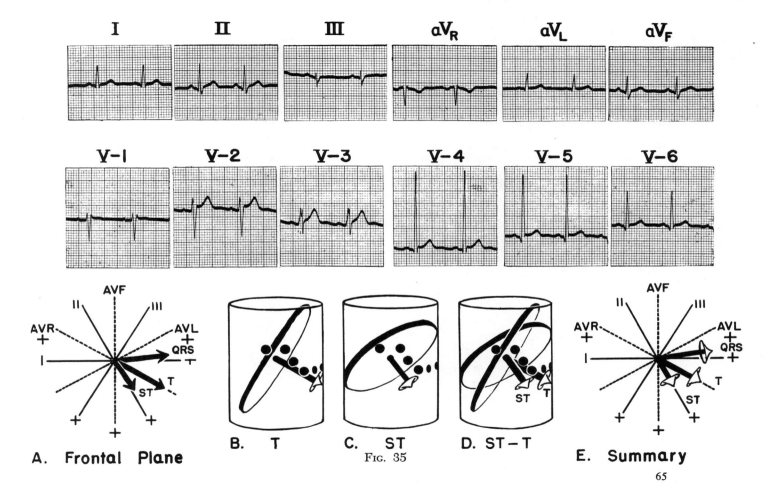

I II III aV_R aV_L aV_F

V-1 V-2 V-3 V-4 V-5 V-6

A. Frontal Plane

B. T

C. ST

D. ST-T

E. Summary

FIG. 35

65

Fig. 36. The electrocardiogram of a normal adult, age 70, illustrating the value of additional precordial leads.

(A) The frontal plane projection of the mean spatial QRS and T vectors. The QRS complex is resultantly zero in Lead aV_F and is larger and positive in Lead I. This enables one to draw the mean QRS vector to the left and parallel to Lead I. The T wave is largest and positive in Lead I and is slightly positive in Lead aV_F. These T wave findings can be represented by a mean T vector 10° to the right of the mean QRS.

(B) The mean spatial QRS vector orientated in the cylindrical replica of the chest. The QRS must be rotated 20° posteriorly because the transitional pathway passes between the electrode positions V-2 and V-3.

(C) Since the T waves are positive in all the routine precordial leads and no "transitional" T wave is present, one can not accurately estimate the degree of anterior T vector rotation. An additional chest lead such as V-3 recorded on the right side of the chest (V-3R) may be helpful. Where the electrode is placed depends on the characteristics of the vector under study. (C) shows the deflection recorded from electrode position V-3R.

(D) The mean spatial T vector oriented in the cylindrical replica of the chest. The mean T vector must be rotated 20° anteriorly because the transitional pathway passes between electrode position V-1 and V-3R.

(E) Final summary figure illustrating a spatial QRS-T angle of 40°. In the elderly person it is not uncommon to see a T vector rotated considerably anteriorly producing a spatial QRS-T angle of 90°.

66

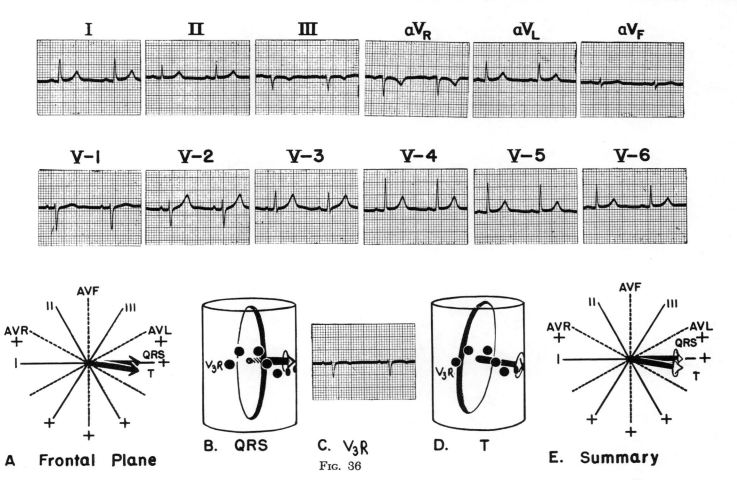

| I | II | III | aV_R | aV_L | aV_F |

| V-1 | V-2 | V-3 | V-4 | V-5 | V-6 |

A. Frontal Plane

B. QRS

C. V₃R

D. T

E. Summary

FIG. 36

CHAPTER THREE

Right and Left Ventricular Hypertrophy

Right Ventricular Hypertrophy

Direction of the Mean and Instantaneous Spatial QRS Vectors. As suggested earlier, the direction of the mean spatial QRS vector indicates the direction of the electrical field in the chest and is governed, for the most part, by the position of the predominant muscle mass. When there is sufficient right ventricular hypertrophy, the mean spatial QRS vector is directed to the right and anteriorly because the right ventricle lies to the right and is anterior to the left ventricle. The amount the mean QRS vector rotates to the right and anteriorly varies greatly from subject to subject. When the mean spatial QRS vector is rotated to the right and anteriorly, the precordial electrode deflections are greatly different from the normal. The R wave is largest in V-1 and becomes progressively smaller in an orderly sequence until it is smallest in V-6, while the S wave is smallest in V-1 but becomes progressively deeper until it is largest in V-6. This is the reverse of what is seen when the mean spatial QRS is normally directed and has been called "reversal of the R/S ratio." The reverse of the R/S ratio is a result of the abnormal QRS loop. In space, the initial instantaneous forces of the QRS loop are directed to the left and anteriorly, the succeeding forces are directed more anteriorly and to the right, and the terminal forces are directed to the right and more posteriorly.

Unfortunately, considerable right ventricular hypertrophy may be present when the mean spatial QRS vector is simply vertical in direction and plumb with the frontal plane, so that the precordial leads are not greatly different from the normal. This is especially true in cases of cor pulmonale resulting from chronic lung disease and in minor degrees of right ventricular hypertrophy resulting from mitral stenosis. Determining right ventricular hypertrophy by studying the direction of the mean spatial QRS vector is fairly reliable in congenital heart disease since it appears to be more strikingly rightward and anteriorly directed. During the neonatal period the mean spatial QRS vector may be directed to the right and anteriorly in the normal subject, indicating right ventricular preponderance which is indeed present. Unfortunately there is no way to separate the normal right ventricular hypertrophy of early life from abnormal right ventricular hypertrophy. This is understandable when one remembers that time must elapse for the myocardium to adapt to the congenital lesion which can in time produce abnormal hypertrophy. When right and left ventricular hypertrophy are present, the mean spatial QRS vector may be entirely normal in direction but increased in magnitude.

The recognition of hypertrophy of the right ventricle from the direction of the mean spatial QRS vector is much more reliable than is the recognition of left ventricular hypertrophy from the direction of the mean spatial QRS vector.

Magnitude of the QRS Complexes. The QRS complexes may or may not be increased in magnitude as compared with normal complexes. Although criteria for right ventricular hypertrophy, utilizing R and S amplitudes, have been suggested and are somewhat helpful, such criteria are not given here for the following reasons: (1) Determining the mean spatial QRS vector position appears to be a more reliable method for recognizing it. (2) The amplitude of a certain deflection not only depends on the actual electrical potential produced by the heart muscle but also varies with electrode distance from the heart. In the child or thin-chested adult, QRS deflections may be large in the chest leads because the electrodes are nearer the heart, whereas chest lead deflections may be small in emphysematous or obese persons even when hypertrophy is present because the distance of the electrodes from the heart is increased.

Duration of the QRS Complexes. The QRS duration may be slightly prolonged but is usually less than .12 second in the adult and less than .10 second in the child.

Direction of the Mean Spatial T Vector. The position of the mean T vector is probably related to the transmyocardial pressure gradient. This pressure gradient depends on the amount of right ventricular pressure and the degree of right ventricular hypertrophy. Frequently this relationship forces the T processes to occur in a manner opposite to usual in the right ventricle and causes the resultant of all T forces to be directed away from the right ventricle. Accordingly, the mean spatial T vector associated with right ventricular hypertrophy is usually directed to the left and is usually flush with the frontal plane or directed a variable number of degrees posteriorly. The spatial QRS-T angle is frequently 150° to 180°.

Direction of the Mean Spatial ST Vector. A measurable ST segment displacement is frequently present. This displacement when illustrated as a spatial vector will usually be directed fairly parallel with the mean spatial T vector. Such an ST vector probably represents the forces of repolarization occurring during the ST interval.

In the electrocardiograms that follow (figs. 37, 38, 39, 40, 41), illustrating right ventricular hypertrophy, it should be noted that the mean QRS vector is usually directed to the right and is either flush with the frontal plane or directed anteriorly. The electrocardiograms have been arranged so that the mean QRS vector is seen to drift farther and farther to the right from tracing to tracing. It is interesting to study the many different deflection contours which result from a slight change in QRS vector position. It should be obvious that when the QRS, ST, and T deflections of twelve electrocardiographic leads are reduced to three spatial vectors, a simpler and more basic electrocardiographic interpretation will result.

Fig. 37. The electrocardiogram of a patient, 35 years of age with mitral stenosis.

(A) The QRS complex is approximately equal and positive in Leads II and III and approximately equal and negative in Lead aV_R and aV_L. The QRS complex is resultantly slightly positive in Lead I. The mean QRS vector is directed downward and located so that a small positive quantity will be projected on Lead I. The ST segment displacement is greatest and negative in Lead II and slightly negative in Lead I. The mean ST vector is directed cephalad and located so that a small negative quantity will be projected on Lead I. The T waves (the last portion of the ST-T segment) are small in the frontal plane and appear to be isoelectric in Lead III. Accordingly, the mean T vector is directed perpendicular to Lead III.

(B), (C), (D) The spatial orientation of the mean QRS, ST, and T vectors. The mean QRS vector is rotated roughly 30° posteriorly because the transitional pathway passes between V-3 and V-4. The mean ST vector is rotated 10° posteriorly because the transitional pathway passes through V-2. Note that the ST segment is elevated in V-1 and depressed in V-3, V-4, V-5, and V-6. The mean T vector is rotated 5° anteriorly because the transitional pathway passes between V-1 and V-2 and is almost resultantly zero in V-1.

(E) Final summary figure. The mean spatial QRS vector is directed vertically and slightly posteriorly. The characteristic electrocardiographic evidence of right ventricular hypertrophy, namely, that the mean QRS vector is directed to the right and anteriorly, is not present here. The mean QRS vector shown above can be perfectly normal or may be present in right ventricular hypertrophy. This is especially true in cases of chronic cor pulmonale and in minor degrees of right ventricular hypertrophy resulting from mitral stenosis. The prominent P waves in the above tracing suggest mitral stenosis or cor pulmonale. The ST and T vectors are the result of digitalis medication. The mean ST vector is fairly large and is directed opposite to the mean QRS vector, while the mean T vector is normally directed but shortened in the frontal plane. The Q-T interval is .32.

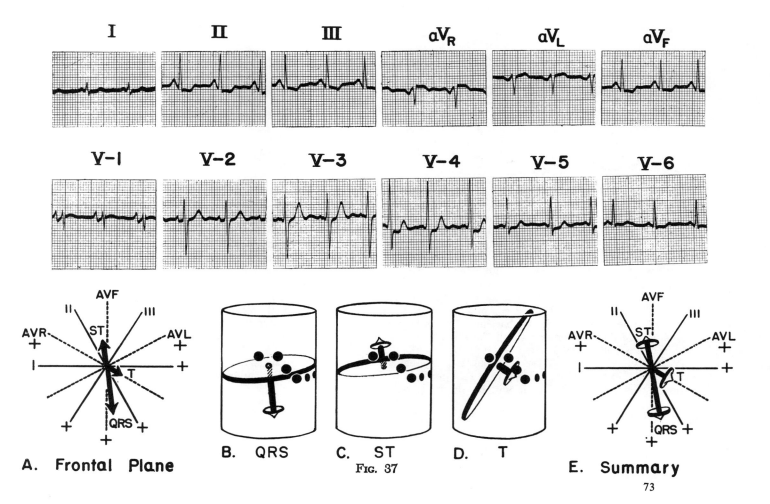

I II III aV_R aV_L aV_F

V-1 V-2 V-3 V-4 V-5 V-6

A. Frontal Plane

B. QRS

C. ST

D. T

Fig. 37

E. Summary

73

Fig. 38. The electrocardiogram of a patient, eight years of age, with pure pulmonary stenosis, illustrating right ventricular hypertrophy.

(A) The QRS complex is approximately equal and positive in Leads II and III, and equal and negative in Leads aV_R and aV_L. The QRS deflection is resultantly slightly negative in Lead I. When the QRS force is represented as a vector, it will be drawn parallel to the positive limb of Lead aV_F but must project a small negative quantity on Lead I. The T wave is largest and positive in Lead II and smallest but negative in Lead aV_L. Accordingly, the mean T vector will be drawn just to the right of the positive limb of Lead II. The ST segment elevation seen in the first complex in Lead III is an artifact due to a wandering baseline. This is known by studying the ST segment in all the other extremity leads and recalling that Leads I + III = II, and aV_R + aV_L + aV_F = 0. The ST segment elevation is greatest in Lead II and therefore the ST vector responsible for the ST segment displacement will be drawn parallel with the positive limb of Lead II. Note that the mean ST vector is relatively parallel with the mean T vector.

(B), (C), (D) The spatial orientation of the QRS, ST, and T vectors. The mean QRS vector is rotated 10° anteriorly because the transitional pathway passes between V-1 and V-2. Actually the QRS complex at V-2 is the only resultantly negative precordial QRS deflection. The mean ST vector is rotated at least 10° anteriorly because the transitional pathway for ST passes through V-1. Since all precordial T waves are positive, the mean T vector is rotated at least 20° anteriorly.

(E) Final summary figure. The mean spatial QRS vector is directed vertically, slightly to the right, and anteriorly. Normal persons may have a mean spatial QRS vector directed just as vertically as in the above case. The differential point lies in the fact that the normal mean spatial QRS vector is directed posteriorly whereas the mean spatial QRS vector shown above is directed anteriorly, indicating right ventricular hypertrophy.

74

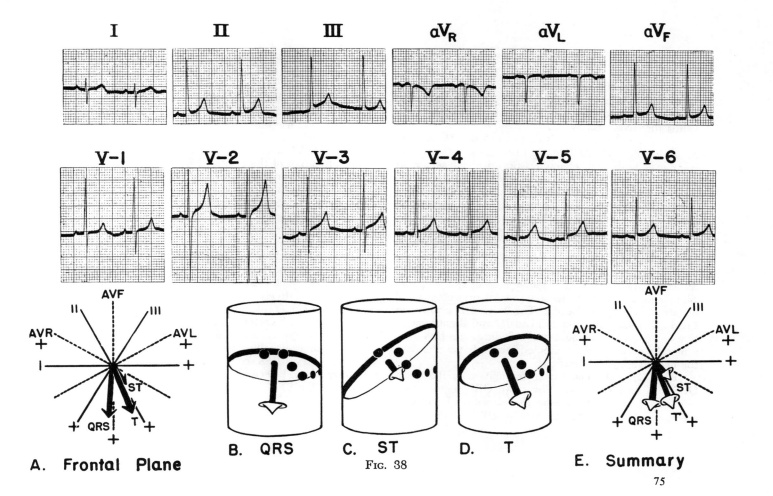

I   II   III   aVR   aVL   aVF

V-1   V-2   V-3   V-4   V-5   V-6

A. Frontal Plane

B. QRS   C. ST   D. T

Fig. 38

E. Summary

75

FIG. 39. The electrocardiogram of a patient, 38 years of age, with interatrial septal defect, illustrating right ventricular hypertrophy.

(A) The QRS complex is largest in Lead III and resultantly slightly negative in Lead aV$_R$. When QRS complexes with such characteristics are represented as a mean vector it will be directed just to the left of the positive limb of Lead III. It is difficult to identify where the ST segment ends and where the T wave begins and the ST-T waves could best be illustrated together as a loop. Considering this difficulty, the ST segment, studied in all extremity leads, appears negative in Leads II and III and just slightly negative in Lead I. A mean vector responsible for the ST segment displacement will be directed parallel with the negative limb of lead aV$_F$ and slightly to the right of that line since it projects a small negative quantity on Lead I. The T wave is positive in Lead I and most negative in Lead III and slightly negative in Lead aV$_R$. These T wave findings can be represented by a mean vector directed relatively parallel with the negative limb of Lead III.

(B), (C), (D) The spatial orientation of the mean QRS, ST, and T vectors. The mean QRS vector is rotated 85° anteriorly because the transitional pathway passes very near electrode V-6. A QRS vector so located will cause almost all anterior chest leads to be resultantly positive. The mean ST vector is tilted 10° posteriorly because the ST segment in V-1 is isoelectric and the remaining ST segments are negative. (The ST segment in V-2 is negative and must have recorded from the negative half of the electrical field. Slight electrode misplacement near electrode position V-2 would alter the ST segment a great deal.) The T wave appears negative in all leads, suggesting that the T vector is tilted 85° posteriorly.

(E) Final summary figure showing the spatial arrangement of the vectors. The mean QRS vector is directed downward, to the right, and is rotated markedly anteriorly while the T vector is rotated 170° away from the mean QRS vector. Frequently a mean ST vector will be seen to be relatively parallel with the mean T vector as in this case. Under such circumstances the T vector is large and the ST vector relatively small while in this case the ST vector is large and the T vector is somewhat smaller than is usually expected. This finding plus a short QT interval (.28 second) and a slightly prolonged P-R interval (.21 second) indicates digitalis effect in addition to the ST-T change of right ventricular hypertrophy.

76

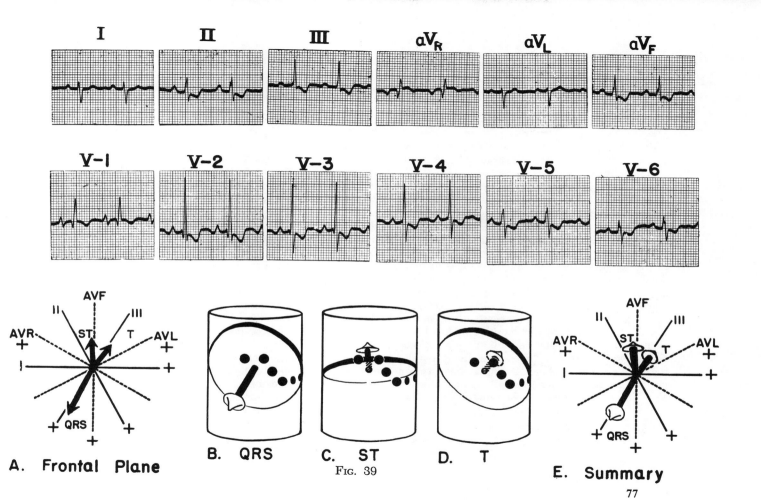

I   II   III   aV_R   aV_L   aV_F

V-1   V-2   V-3   V-4   V-5   V-6

A. Frontal Plane   B. QRS   C. ST   D. T   E. Summary

Fig. 39

77

FIG. 40. The electrocardiogram of a patient 30 years of age with mitral stenosis, illustrating right ventricular hypertrophy.

(A) The QRS complex is large and positive in Lead III and large and negative in Lead aV_L. The QRS complex is resultantly slightly positive in Lead II. Accordingly, the mean QRS vector is relatively parallel with the negative limb of Lead aV_L but is directed so that it projects a small positive quantity on Lead II. It is difficult to identify where the ST segment ends and where the T wave begins. The ST segment appears largest and negative in Lead III, slightly negative in Lead II, and isoelectric in Lead aV_R. The mean ST vector is therefore directed parallel to the negative limb of Lead III. The T wave is largest and positive in Lead I, slightly positive in Lead II, and resultantly zero in Lead aV_F. The mean T vector is directed relatively parallel with the positive limb of Lead I. The P wave is large and positive in Lead II and is small and negative in Lead aV_L. The mean P vector is therefore directed just to the right of the positive limb of Lead II.

(B), (C), (D) The spatial orientation of the mean QRS, ST, T, and P vectors. The mean QRS vector is directed 20° anteriorly because the transitional pathway passes through V-3. The mean ST vector is directed 20° to 30° posteriorly and the mean T vector is directed 20° posteriorly. The mean P vector is directed 5° posteriorly because the transitional pathway for the mean P vector passes very near V-2. The large P wave deflections indicate atrial enlargement.

(E) Final summary figure showing the spatial arrangement of the vectors. The mean QRS vector is directed to the right and anteriorly indicating right ventricular hypertrophy. Tremendous P waves, as illustrated in this tracing, usually indicate left atrial enlargement. The rather large ST vector associated with a relatively small T vector and a short Q-T interval (.28 second) suggests digitalis effect. Note that an abnormally wide QRS-T angle can be recognized in this case even though digitalis effect is present.

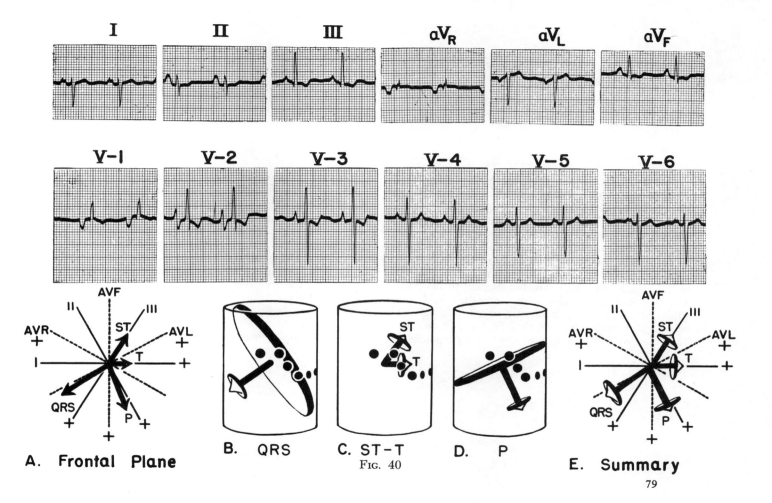

I II III aV_R aV_L aV_F

V-1 V-2 V-3 V-4 V-5 V-6

A. Frontal Plane

B. QRS

C. ST-T

D. P

FIG. 40

E. Summary

79

FIG. 41. The electrocardiogram of a patient, three years of age, with tetralogy of Fallot, illustrating right ventricular hypertrophy.

(A) The QRS complexes vary greatly with respiration but when long strips are studied, it becomes apparent that the QRS complex is smallest and slightly negative on Lead aV_F, resultantly zero on Lead III and negative on Leads I and II. Such QRS complexes can be illustrated by a mean vector directed parallel to Lead aV_R. The T wave also varies with respiration and when studied in a long strip is slightly negative in Lead III and slightly positive in Lead aV_F. Such a T wave can be illustrated by a vector drawn between a perpendicular to Lead III and a perpendicular to Lead aV_F.

(B), (C) The spatial orientation of the mean QRS and T vectors. The mean QRS vector is rotated 5° posteriorly because the transitional pathway passes between V-1 and V-2. The T vector is flush with the frontal plane because the transitional pathway passes between the V-1 and V-2 position.

(D) Final summary figure showing the spatial arrangement of the vectors. The mean QRS vector is rotated slightly posteriorly. When the mean QRS vector is rotated *markedly* to the right, slightly posteriorly directed QRS vectors may be encountered but it is rare for the displacement to be more than 5°.

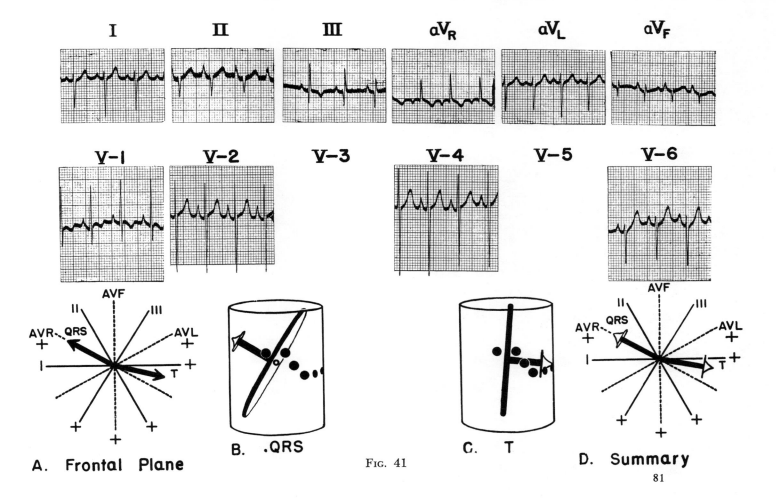

I II III aV_R aV_L aV_F

V-1 V-2 V-3 V-4 V-5 V-6

A. Frontal Plane

B. .QRS

C. T

D. Summary

Fig. 41

81

Left Ventricular Hypertrophy

Direction of the Mean and Instantaneous Spatial QRS Vectors. As stated previously in the discussion of right ventricular hypertrophy, the mean spatial QRS vector points toward the area of predominant muscle mass. Accordingly, in left ventricular hypertrophy, the mean QRS vector is often directed farther to the left and more posteriorly than normally. However, in many instances there may be no deviation in direction from the normal. In certain individuals with narrow body builds so that the heart occupies a vertical position, the left ventricle lies more vertically, and with hypertrophy the mean QRS vector is increased in magnitude but vertical in direction.

The initial instantaneous forces of the QRS loop are usually so directed that the QRS loop is inscribed in a counter-clockwise direction when viewed in the frontal plane. Usually the early forces of the QRS loop project a negative quantity on Lead I producing a narrow Q wave in this lead. Often left ventricular hypertrophy and left bundle branch block are quite similar and a small Q wave in Lead I suggests that the abnormality is left ventricular hypertrophy. An exception to this is left bundle branch block in the presence of septal infarction, since a Q wave can occur in Lead I under such circumstances. On rare occasions the entire QRS loop may rotate so far to the left that a QS deflection is written in Lead III and aV$_F$. In such a case it may be impossible to exclude an old posterior infarction superimposed on the electrocardiographic abnormality of left ventricular hypertrophy. When viewed in space, the initial forces of the QRS loop are usually anteriorly directed and are never posterior to the mean spatial QRS vector. At times the entire QRS loop may be so posteriorly rotated that Leads V-1, V-2, and V-3 may record QS deflections. In such a case the absent R waves suggest anterior myocardial infarction and at times it may be impossible to state that such has not been superimposed on the abnormalities of left ventricular hypertrophy.

Magnitude of the QRS Complexes. When the ventricular muscle increases in thickness, the mean QRS vector, representing all the QRS vectors, is increased in magnitude. When the deflection magnitude is studied, one should recall that electrode distance is a very important factor. For instance QRS deflections may be large in thin-chested persons with no cardiac hypertrophy but small in thick-chested persons even when hypertrophy is present. If the chest wall is thick and the QRS deflection in V-5 or V-6 is more than 25 mm, it is considered suggestive of left ventricular hypertrophy and may be the only electrocardiographic evidence of this condition. Many cases of left ventricular hypertrophy are not associated with increased QRS voltage and the absence of such a finding should not be used as evidence against hypertrophy.

Duration of the QRS Complexes. The QRS duration, though often normal, may be prolonged to .11 or even .12 second. Most electrocardiographers state that ventricular hypertrophy alone will not prolong the QRS duration beyond .12 second.

Direction of the Mean Spatial T Vector. As in right ventricular hypertrophy the direction of the mean spatial T vector is probably related to the transmyocardial pressure gradient for the T is generated when the heart is in the contracted state. Two of the governing factors appear to be the amount of left ventricular systolic pressure and the degree of left ventricular hypertrophy. Frequently in left ventricular hypertrophy this relationship is such that T processes in the left ventricle are produced in a manner opposite to the usual manner and the resultant of all T forces is directed away from the left ventricle. Accordingly, in left ventricular hypertrophy the mean T vector is frequently directed to the right and anteriorly. This produces an abnormally wide spatial QRS-T angle. The spatial QRS-T angle may, in the beginning, be entirely normal but with the passage of time the angle will usually gradually become wider and finally become 160° to 180°. The "strain" pattern has been applied to the electrocardiographic findings of ventricular hypertrophy associated with a QRS-T angle of 160° to 180°. The term "strain" has created confusion in the past and therefore is not used in this book.

Direction of the Mean Spatial ST Vector. ST segment displacement is frequently present and can be represented by a vector. The mean spatial ST vector of left ventricular hypertrophy is nearly parallel with the mean spatial T vector. Such an ST vector probably represents forces of repolarization occurring during the ST interval. Occasionally an abnormally directed ST vector may appear before the T wave abnormality occurs.

The following electrocardiograms (figs. 42, 43, 44, 45) have been arranged so that the mean QRS vector is seen to drift farther and farther to the left from tracing to tracing.

Fig. 42. The electrocardiogram of a patient, 32 years of age, with rheumatic calcific aortic stenosis, illustrating left ventricular hypertrophy.

(A) The QRS complex is largest in Lead II, slightly positive in Lead I and negative in Lead aV$_L$. QRS complexes of this nature can be represented by a mean vector directed to the right of the positive limb of Lead II. The T wave is slightly negative in Lead I, large and negative in Leads II, III and aV$_F$, and positive in Lead aV$_L$. Accordingly, the mean T vector is directed to the right of the negative limb of Lead aV$_F$ but to the left of a perpendicular to Lead aV$_L$.

(B), (C) The spatial orientation of the mean QRS and T vectors. The mean QRS is rotated 50° posteriorly because the transitional pathway passes between the V-4 and V-5 position. The mean T vector is tilted 50° anteriorly because the transitional pathway passes between the V-4 and V-5 position. Note the increased magnitude of the QRS complexes.

(D) Final summary figure showing the spatial arrangement of the vectors. The mean QRS vector is directed downward and posteriorly and the mean T vector is directed to the right and anteriorly. The spatial QRS-T angle is 180°. These findings are characteristic of left ventricular hypertrophy associated with an abnormally wide QRS-T angle. The mean QRS is vertically directed and may be related to the thin, long-chested, build of the patient.

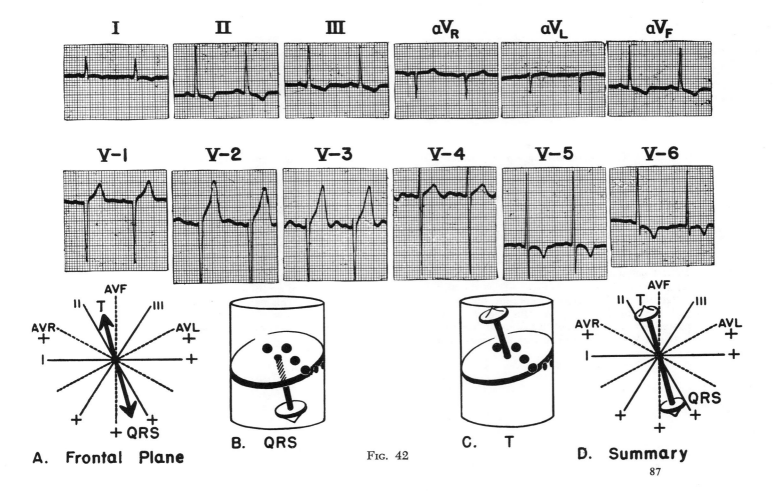

I II III aV_R aV_L aV_F

V-1 V-2 V-3 V-4 V-5 V-6

A. Frontal Plane

B. QRS

C. T

D. Summary

F_IG. 42

Fig. 43. The electrocardiogram of a patient, 51 years of age, with essential hypertension, illustrating left ventricular hypertrophy.

(A) The QRS complex is resultantly zero in Lead III and positive in Leads I and II. The mean QRS vector is therefore directed perpendicular to Lead III. The T wave is large and negative in Lead I and slightly positive in Lead aV_F. The mean T vector is therefore directed relatively parallel with the negative limb of the Lead I axis but must project a small positive quantity on Lead aV_F.

(B), (C) The spatial orientation of the mean QRS and T vectors. The mean QRS vector is rotated 30° posteriorly because the transitional pathway passes between V-3 and V-4. The mean T vector is tilted 30° anteriorly because the transitional pathway passes between V-3 and V-4.

(D) Final summary figure showing the spatial arrangement of the vectors. The QRS voltage is large. The mean QRS vector is directed to the left and posteriorly and the mean T vector is directed to the right and anteriorly. Because the QRS and T vectors are directed in such a manner the QRS complex is upright in Lead I and V-6 and the T wave is inverted in Lead I and V-6. This "pattern" has been recognized as indicating left ventricular hypertrophy for years. The spatial QRS-T angle is 150°. This patient was on digitalis but its effect is masked because of the ST and T changes of left ventricular hypertrophy. (Digitalis effect will be discussed later.)

88

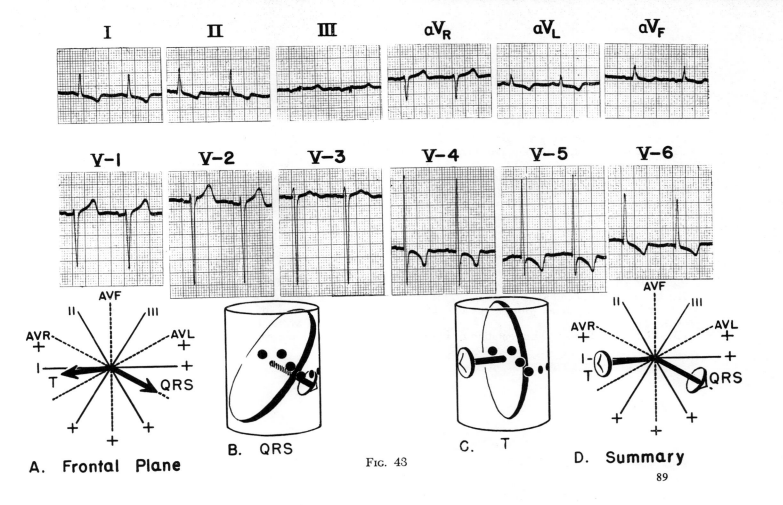

I	II	III	aV_R	aV_L	aV_F

V-1	V-2	V-3	V-4	V-5	V-6

A. Frontal Plane

B. QRS

C. T

D. Summary

Fig. 43

89

FIG. 44. The electrocardiogram of a patient, 61 years of age, with essential hypertension, illustrating left ventricular hypertrophy.

(A) The QRS complex is large and positive in Lead I, resultantly positive in Lead II, and resultantly negative in Lead aV_F. The mean QRS vector is therefore directed relatively parallel with the positive limb of Lead I but must be directed slightly cephalad in order to project a slightly negative quantity on Lead aV_F. The T wave is large and negative in Lead I and flat in Lead II. The mean T vector is therefore directed perpendicular to Lead II. The ST segment displacement is greatest in Lead I and least in Lead aV_F. Accordingly, the mean ST vector is directed parallel with the negative limb of Lead I.

(B), (C), (D) The spatial orientation of the mean QRS, ST, and T vectors. The mean QRS vector is directed 20° posteriorly because the transitional pathway passes between V-2 and V-3. The mean ST vector is directed 30° anteriorly because the transitional pathway passes between V-3 and V-4. The mean T vector is directed 30° anteriorly because the transitional pathway passes between V-3 and V-4. Note that the mean spatial ST vector is relatively parallel with the mean spatial T vector.

(E) Final summary figure showing the spatial arrangement of the vectors. The mean QRS vector is directed to the left and posteriorly and the mean T vector is directed to the right and anteriorly. The QRS voltage is increased and the spatial QRS-T angle is 175°. The mean ST vector is relatively parallel to the mean T vector and represents forces of repolarization.

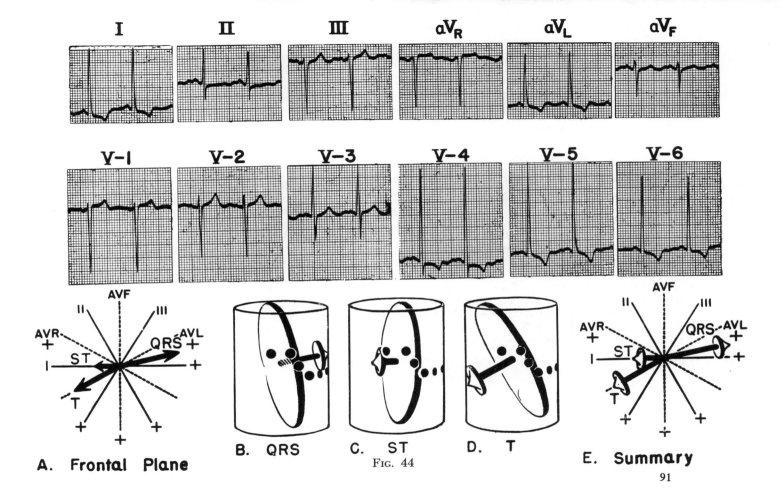

I	II	III	aV$_R$	aV$_L$	aV$_F$

V-1	V-2	V-3	V-4	V-5	V-6

A. Frontal Plane B. QRS C. ST D. T E. Summary

Fig. 44

91

Fig. 45. The electrocardiogram of a patient, 15 years of age, with coarctation of the aorta, illustrating left ventricular hypertrophy.

(A) The QRS complex is largest and negative in Lead III and slightly negative in Lead II. QRS complexes of this nature can be represented by a mean vector directed just cephalad to a perpendicular to Lead II and pointing toward the positive pole of aV_L. The T wave is smallest and slightly positive in Lead II and slightly negative in Lead aV_F. Accordingly, the mean T vector is located between the positive limb of Lead I and the positive limb of Lead aV_L.

(B), (C) The spatial orientation of the mean QRS and T vectors. The mean QRS vector is rotated 50° posteriorly because the transitional pathway passes between V-4 and V-5. The mean T vector is rotated 85° anteriorly because the transitional pathway lies very near V-6. A mean T vector in this position will be foreshortened in the frontal plane and large in the anterior precordial leads.

(D) Final summary figure showing the spatial arrangement of the vectors. The mean QRS vector is directed markedly leftward and posteriorly. Note that the frontal plane projection of the QRS-T angle is entirely normal but that the spatial QRS-T angle is roughly 135°.

92

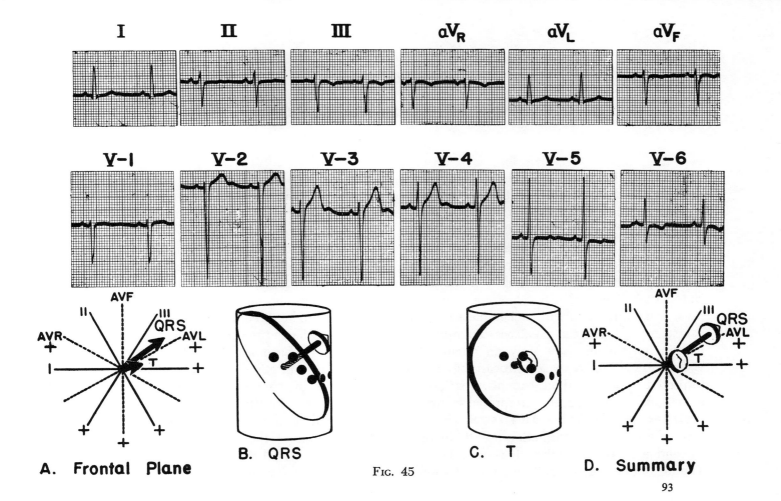

I II III aV_R aV_L aV_F

V-1 V-2 V-3 V-4 V-5 V-6

A. Frontal Plane

B. QRS

C. T

D. Summary

Fig. 45

93

CHAPTER FOUR

Myocardial Infarction

There are three electrocardiographic abnormalities resulting from an acute myocardial infarction: (1) an abnormally directed mean spatial vector for the initial .04 second of the QRS cycle, (2) a prominent mean spatial ST vector, and (3) an abnormally directed mean spatial T vector. From the outset it should be stated that a patient may experience an acute myocardial infarction with a characteristic clinical story and yet the electrocardiogram may remain normal, or show only an abnormal T vector. Accordingly, the electrocardiogram, interpreted by any method, cannot substitute for a well taken and properly interpreted history.

(1) The Mean Spatial Initial .04 Vector. The dead zone of a myocardial infarction usually involves the endocardial half of the left ventricular wall. The dead area is electrically inert and therefore cannot undergo depolarization or repolarization. Because the dead area does not contribute forces during the early period of ventricular depolarization, the unopposed electrical forces generated in the diametrically opposite region of the heart dominate the electrical field during this early period. Accordingly, the initial portion of the QRS loop becomes deformed because the initial forces tend to be directed away from the area of dead tissue. Since the early forces of ventricular depolarization become abnormally directed after myocardial infarction, one can identify such dead areas by studying the deformity of the initial .04 second of the QRS loop. As a rule it is not necessary to plot the entire spatial QRS loop, since calculating the mean spatial initial .04 vector is usually all that is needed to identify a myocardial dead zone. This vector, representing the resultant of all the instantaneous vectors generated during the initial .04 second of the QRS loop, tends to be directed away from the area of dead tissue. The position of this vector and its relationship to the mean spatial QRS vector must be identified. At times, however, in unusual tracings, it is desirable to construct the entire QRS loop as seen in the frontal and transverse planes.

Since the diagnosis of myocardial dead zone depends on identifying an abnormality of the QRS loop or an abnormally directed mean spatial initial .04 vector, it is desirable to restate the characteristics of the normal QRS loop and normal mean .04 vector. The normal QRS loop is narrow and elongate. In the normal subject a line drawn through the termini of the instantaneous vectors passes in a smooth and orderly manner to encompass the mean spatial QRS vector. At times, especially when viewed in the frontal plane, a crisscrossed figure results. When viewed in the frontal plane in the normal subject, the mean initial .04 vector tends to be nearly parallel with the mean QRS vector and usually lies between the positive limb of Lead

aV_F and the positive limb of Lead I. It is usually located to the right of a markedly leftward mean QRS vector, to the left of a vertically located mean QRS vector, but may be found on either side of a mean QRS vector located in the intermediate zone. When viewed in space, the mean spatial initial .04 vector is always directed anterior to the mean spatial QRS vector. The QRS loop, viewed in the transverse plane, begins in the approximate center of the chest and tends to rotate leftward and anteriorly, and then posteriorly.

A myocardial dead zone then may cause a deformity of the QRS loop and an abnormally directed initial .04 vector. The location of the area of electrically inert tissue determines the type of QRS loop deformity and the particular direction the initial .04 vector takes. The degree of QRS loop deformity and the magnitude of the initial .04 vector is roughly proportional to the size of the dead area. An abnormal QRS loop deformity or an abnormally directed mean initial .04 vector may not occur if the dead area is small or if the diametrically opposite ventricular myocardium is dead and unable to generate electrical forces.

95

When a myocardial infarct involves the inferior or diaphragmatic portion of the left ventricle, the initial instantaneous vectors of the QRS loop and the mean initial .04 vector will be directed toward the left shoulder since they tend to be directed away from the area of dead muscle. In such a case the mean initial .04 vector is usually directed to the left of a moderately leftward mean QRS vector and will be directed 90° or more to the left of an intermediate or vertically directed mean QRS vector. When the initial portion of the QRS loop is directed as described, an R wave will be recorded in Lead I and aV_L and a Q wave of .03 to .04 second in duration will be recorded in Leads II, III, and aV_F. This pattern has been utilized for years to identify an infarction of the inferior and diaphragmatic wall of the left ventricle (see figs. 58 and 70A). One should not diagnose infarction if only the initial .01 or .02 QRS vector is directed toward the left shoulder and the Q wave in Leads II and III is .02 second or less in duration, since this may occur normally. At times, when the infarction is large and involves almost the entire thickness of the ventricular wall, the entire QRS loop may rotate to the left, causing QS deflections to be recorded in Leads III and aV_F.

Infarction of the anterior and lateral wall of the left ventricle causes the initial instantaneous vectors of the QRS loop and the mean initial .04 vector to be directed to the right and posteriorly. In such a case the mean initial .04 vector may be directed abnormally to the right of a vertically directed mean QRS vector or more than 90° to the right of a leftward mean QRS vector. When the initial stroke of the QRS loop is so directed, a Q wave will be recorded in Leads I and aV_L and an R wave will be recorded in Leads II, III, and aV_F. This pattern has been called anterior or anterolateral myocardial infarction. An infarct located in the anterolateral region may cause the transverse plane QRS loop to rotate to the right and posteriorly, rather than to the left and posteriorly as it does normally. This QRS loop abnormality causes R waves to be recorded in the right precordial leads and abnormal Q waves to be recorded in the left precordial leads. When the anterolateral infarct is large and involves almost the entire thickness of the muscle wall, the entire QRS loop may be rotated to the right, causing QS deflections to be recorded in Leads I and aV$_L$ (see fig. 65).

When the anterior free wall and adjacent septal portion of the left ventricle are the site of infarction, the initial instantaneous vectors of the QRS loop and the mean initial .04 vector will be directed abnormally posteriorly. The abnormally posteriorly directed initial stroke of the QRS loop can be identified when the mean initial .04 vector is directed posterior to the mean QRS vector. When the infarct is extensive, the initial .04 vector may be directed toward the negative pole of Leads V-1, V-2, V-3, and V-4. In other words, a large anterior infarct can cause QS complexes to be recorded in Leads V-1, V-2, V-3, and V-4 (see figs. 66 and 70C). QS complexes may be recorded in V-1 in normal subjects and QS complexes may be recorded in V-1, V-2, and V-3 in cases of left ventricular hypertrophy, but it is rare for all the instantaneous vectors generated during the initial .04 second of the QRS cycle to be directed so posteriorly that V-1, V-2, V-3, and V-4 record no R waves. There may be little if any abnormality of the frontal plane

QRS loop but usually, when the infarct is large and extends to the lateral wall, the loop abnormality described in the previous paragraph will be present.

When a relatively small anteroseptal infarct occurs, the initial instantaneous forces of the QRS loop are directed posteriorly and little frontal plane abnormality occurs. In this case the mean initial .04 vector is frequently directed abnormally posteriorly to the mean QRS vector. At times, with such an infarct, the abnormality may involve the forces generated during the initial .02 second rather than those generated during the initial .04 second. Here it is useful to construct the transverse plane QRS loop and visualize the QRS loop deformity (see figs. 61 and 70B, figs. 68 and 70D). This type of abnormality can be recognized quickly without constructing the entire QRS loop by identifying an initial instantaneous vector directed posteriorly to the subsequent instantaneous vector regardless of the duration of the vectors, since this rarely occurs normally. This type of QRS loop abnormality is identified empirically by noting the absence of an R wave in Leads V-1 and V-2 and a small Q followed by R and S waves in Lead V-3.

When the left ventricular apex is the site of an infarction, little QRS abnormality, other than reduced magnitude, results. This is because the myocardium generating a large portion of the normal initial forces is still intact and because there is little ventricular muscle diametrically opposite to the cardiac apex (see fig. 50). If the apical infarct is large and properly located, the mean initial .04 vector may be directed to the right and at times toward the right shoulder, producing Q waves in Leads I, II, and occasionally Lead III.

The various directions the mean spatial initial .04 vector is caused to take as a result of myocardial infarcts located in various positions in the heart will be illustrated. Since most infarcts occur in the left ventricle and interventricular septum, only these portions of the heart need to be shown when discussing and diagramming infarction. Fig. 46 illustrates the left ventricle and interventricular septum detached from the atria and right ventricle. This diagram was designed to be reasonably accurate from an anatomic standpoint after Grant had dissected ten hearts. The anatomic landmarks were established by preserving the longitudinal, vertical, and

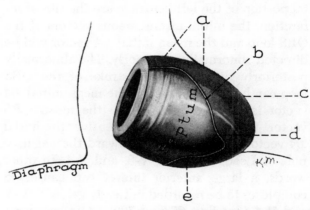

FIG. 46. Diagram illustrating the left ventricle and interventricular septum detached from the atria and right ventricle. (The mitral orifice has been omitted in order to simplify the drawing.) (A) Superior free wall of the left ventricle. (B) Pathway of the anterior descending coronary artery marks the edge of right ventricular contact and hence the anterior edge of septum. (Note that the septum is not flat.) (C) Lateral free wall of the left ventricle. (D) Anterior free wall of the left ventricle. (E) Diaphragmatic free wall of the left ventricle. (Drawn after studying the data of Dr. Robert Grant.)

horizontal axes of the heart in a fixed place in the body before examination. Note especially that the septum is not flat and that a portion of the free wall of the left ventricle lies on the diaphragm. Figs. 47 through 54 illustrate infarcts located in different regions of the left ventricle. Part A of each figure indicates the location of the myocardial infarction. One should recall that the dead zone usually involves the endocardial half of the ventricular wall but in order to simplify the diagrams it was necessary to indicate the location of the dead zone by a thin endocardial disk. A mean initial .04 vector is drawn opposite the dead area to indicate the forces generated by the unopposed diametrically opposite ventricular muscle. The last four figures illustrate the zone of injury and ischemia as well as the dead zone. Part B of each figure shows the mean spatial initial .04 vector transposed to the center of the hexaxial reference system. From this diagram one can see how Q waves and R waves are produced in the extrem-ity leads by studying the projection of the vector on the extremity lead axes. The last four figures also show the frontal plane projection of the mean spatial ST and T vectors. Part C of each diagram illustrates the position of the spatial .04 vector in a cylindrical replica of the chest. From this figure one can study the projection of the mean initial .04 vector on the precordial lead axes.

At times the electrocardiographic localization of a myocardial infarct will not coincide with pathologic localization. One difficulty arises from the fact that the vectors resulting from a myocardial infarction in a vertical heart may project on the routine leads in quite a different manner to the vectors of a similarly located infarction in a horizontal heart. Another reason for the lack of perfect parallelism in electrocardiographic and pathologic localization is the fact that the electrocardiogram reflects electrical death while the pathologist studies the morphologic evidences of necrosis.

FIG. 47. (A) The dead zone of a myocardial infarction is located in the inferior or diaphragmatic surface of the left ventricle. The lower part of the interventricular septum is also frequently involved. The electrical forces generated by the muscle of the diametrically opposite wall dominate the electrical field during the initial .04 second of the QRS cycle and the mean initial .04 vector is directed away from the area of dead tissue.

(B) The mean initial .04 vector is treated as though it originates in the center of the chest and the hexaxial reference system has been superimposed. This enables one to study the projection of the mean initial .04 vector on the extremity lead axes. In this case a Q wave will be written in Leads II, III, aV$_F$, and an R wave will be written in Leads I, aV$_R$, and aV$_L$. This type of myocardial infarction is usually called a posterior infarction.

(C) This figure illustrates how the mean initial .04 vector shown in (A) will influence the precordial leads. In this case there will be initial R waves in all the precordial leads.

100

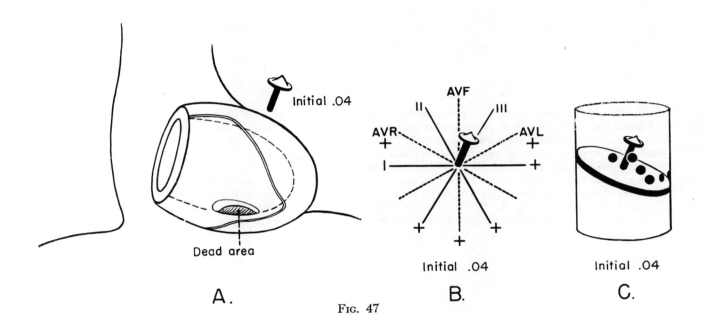

Initial .04

Dead area

A.

AVF

II III

AVR AVL
+ +

I +

+
+ +

Initial .04

B.

Initial .04

C.

Fig. 47

FIG. 48. (A) The dead zone of a myocardial infarction is located on the inferior and posterior surface of the left ventricle. The electrical forces generated by the diametrically opposite part of the heart dominate the electrical field during the initial .04 second of the QRS cycle and the mean initial .04 vector is directed away from the area of inert tissue. (B) The mean initial .04 vector is treated as though it originates in the center of the chest and the hexaxial reference system has been superimposed. This enables one to study the projection of the mean initial .04 vector on the extremity lead axes. In this case a Q wave will be recorded on Leads II, III, aV_F, and aV_R, and an R wave will be recorded in Leads I and aV_L. (C) This figure illustrates how the mean initial .04 vector shown in (A) will influence the precordial leads. In this case initial R waves will be recorded in all the precordial leads.

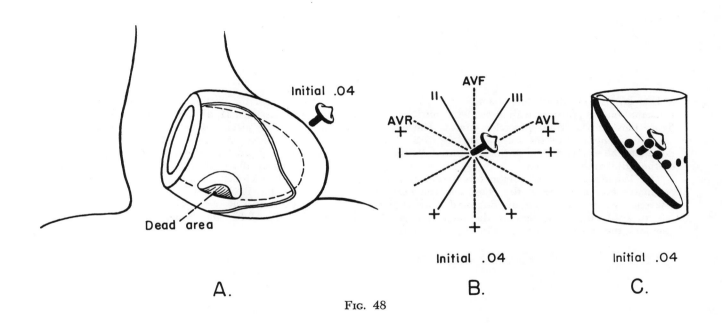

Initial .04

Dead area

AVF

AVR

II   III

AVL

I

Initial .04

A.

B.

C.

Initial .04

Initial .04

Fig. 48

FIG. 49. (A) The dead zone of a myocardial infarction is located on the posterior wall of the left ventricle. This figure illustrates a "true" posterior infarct. The electrical forces generated by the anterior surface of the heart dominate the electrical field during the initial .04 second of the QRS cycle.

(B) The mean initial .04 vector is treated as though it originates in the center of the chest and the hexaxial reference system has been superimposed. This enables one to study the projection of the mean spatial .04 vector on the extremity lead axes. In this case the frontal plane projection of the vector is quite small, producing an R wave in Leads I, II, aV_F, and aV_L, and a Q wave in Lead aV_R. The mean .04 vector is perpendicular to Lead III, and therefore the initial .04 second of the QRS complex in Lead III will be resultantly zero.

(C) This figure illustrates how the mean initial .04 vector shown in (A) will influence the precordial leads. In this case initial R waves will be recorded in all the precordial leads and at times the R wave in the right precordial leads will be quite large.

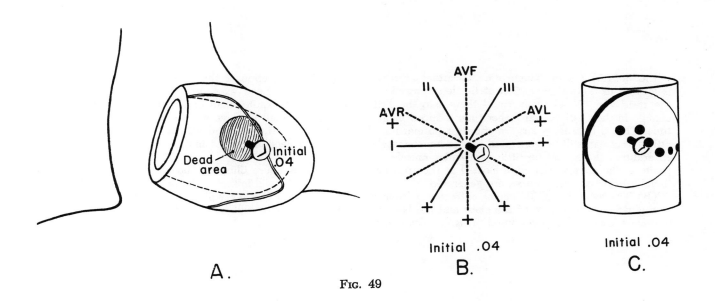

Dead area

Initial .04

A.

AVF

II   III

AVR   AVL
+   +

I   +

+   +

+

Initial .04

B.

Initial .04

C.

Fig. 49

FIG. 50. (A) The dead zone of a myocardial infarction is located in the apical portion of the left ventricle. If the dead zone is relatively small there may be little change in the QRS contour other than reduced magnitude. This is because a large number of normal initial QRS forces can still be generated by the intact muscle. In addition there may be little ventricular muscle opposite to the area of infarction located at the apex and therefore few opposing forces are generated.

(B) The mean initial .04 vector is treated as though it originates in the center of the chest and the hexaxial reference system is superimposed. This enables one to study the projection of the mean initial .04 vector on the extremity Lead axes. In this case the initial .04 vector will be quite small and is directed in a normal manner. A small Q wave will be recorded in Lead III but Leads I, II, aV_L, and aV_F will record a resultant positive deflection for the first .04 second of the QRS cycle.

(C) This figure illustrates how the mean .04 vector shown in (A) will influence the precordial leads. In this case an initial Q wave will be recorded in Lead I and positive R waves will be recorded in Leads V-2, V-3, V-4, V-5, and V-6.

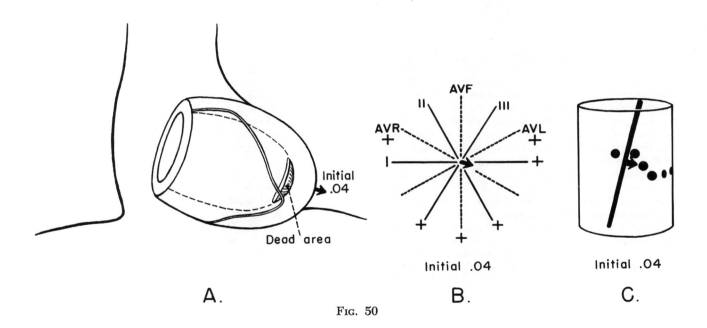

Initial
.04

Dead area

AVF

II   III

AVR   AVL
+   +

I   +

+   +

+

Initial .04

Initial .04

A.

Fig. 50

B.

C.

FIG. 51. (A) The myocardial infarction is located in the lateral portion of the left ventricle. The electrical forces generated in the opposite portion of the heart dominate the electrical field during the initial .04 second of the QRS cycle and the mean initial .04 vector is directed away from the dead tissue. The area of dead tissue is surrounded by an area of myocardial injury which is located predominantly in the epicardial region of the left ventricle. The mean ST vector will be directed toward the area of epicardial injury. The area of dead and injured tissue is surrounded by an area of epicardial ischemia. The mean T vector will be directed away from the area of epicardial ischemia.

(B) The mean initial .04, ST, and T vectors are treated as though they originate in the center of the chest and the hexaxial reference system has been superimposed. This enables one to study the projection of the vectors on the extremity lead axes. In this case a Q wave will be recorded in Leads I and aV_L and an R wave will be recorded in Leads II, III, and aV_F. The mean initial .04 vector is perpendicular to Lead aV_R and therefore the initial .04 second of the QRS complex in Lead aV_R will be resultantly zero. The ST segment will be elevated in Leads I and aV_L and depressed in Leads II, III, aV_F, and aV_R. The T wave will be inverted in Leads I and aV_L and upright in Leads II, III, aV_F, and aV_R.

(C) This figure illustrates how the mean initial .04 vector shown in (A) will influence the precordial leads. In this case a Q wave will be recorded in Leads V-2, V-3, V-4, V-5, and V-6. Although it is not illustrated, the ST segment would be elevated in Leads V-2, V-3, V-4, V-5, and V-6 and depressed in Lead V-1. The T wave would be inverted in V-2, V-3, V-4, V-5, V-6, and upright in Lead V-1.

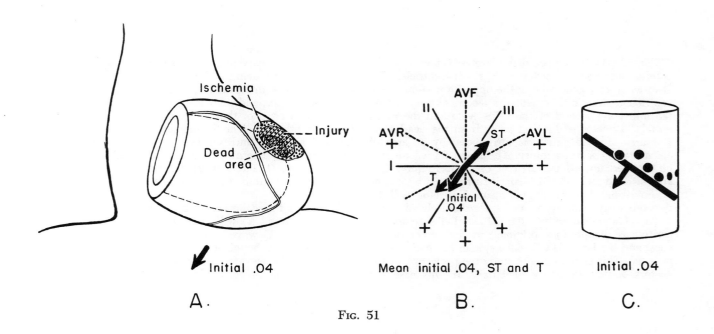

Ischemia

Injury

Dead area

Initial .04

A.

AVF

II   III

AVR   ST   AVL

+   +

I   +

T

Initial .04

+   +

+

Mean initial .04, ST and T

B.

Initial .04

C.

Fig. 51

109

Fig. 52. (A) The myocardial infarction is located in the anterior and septal portion of the left ventricle. The electrical forces generated in the opposite portion of the ventricular muscle dominate the electrical field during the initial .04 second of the QRS cycle and the mean initial .04 vector is directed away from the dead area. The area of dead muscle is surrounded by an area of epicardial myocardial injury. The mean ST vector will be directed toward the area of epicardial injury. The area of dead and injured tissue is surrounded by a zone of epicardial ischemia. The mean T vector will be directed away from the area of epicardial ischemia.

(B) The mean initial .04, ST, and T vectors are treated as though they originate in the center of the chest and the hexaxial reference system has been superimposed. This enables one to study the projection of the vectors on the extremity lead axes. In this case the frontal plane projection of the mean initial .04 vector is quite small, producing a Q wave in Leads I and aV$_L$, and an R wave in Leads III, aV$_F$, and aV$_R$. The mean .04 vector is perpendicular to Lead II and therefore the initial .04 second of the QRS complex in Lead II will be resultantly zero. The ST segment will be elevated in Leads I and aV$_L$ and will be depressed in Leads III, aV$_F$, and aV$_R$. There will be no ST segment displacement in Lead II. The T wave will be inverted in Leads I and aV$_L$ and will be upright in Leads II, III, aV$_F$, and aV$_R$.

(C) This figure illustrates how the mean initial .04 vector shown in (A) will influence the precordial leads. In this case a Q wave will be recorded in all the precordial leads. Although it is not illustrated the ST segment would be elevated and the T waves would be inverted in all the precordial leads.

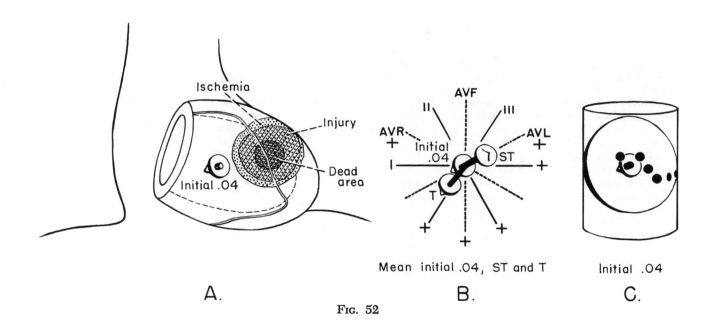

A.

B.

Mean initial .04, ST and T

C.

Initial .04

Fig. 52

111

FIG. 53. (A) The myocardial infarction is located in the anterior, lateral, and septal portion of the left ventricle. The electrical forces generated in the opposite portion of the heart dominate the electrical field during the initial .04 second of the QRS cycle and the mean initial .04 vector is directed away from the dead zone. The area of dead tissue is surrounded by an area of epicardial myocardial injury and the ST vector will be directed toward the area of epicardial injury. Surrounding the latter area is an area of epicardial myocardial ischemia. The mean T vector will be directed away from the area of epicardial ischemia.

(B) The mean initial .04, ST, and T vectors are treated as though they originate in the center of the chest and the hexaxial reference system has been superimposed. This enables one to study the projection of the vectors on the extremity lead axes. In this case a Q wave will be recorded in Leads I, aV_L, and aV_R and an R wave will be recorded in Leads II, III, aV_F. The ST segment will be elevated in Leads I and aV_L and depressed in Leads II, III, aV_F, and aV_R. The T wave will be inverted in Leads I and aV_L, resultantly zero in Lead aV_R and upright in Leads II, III, and aV_F.

(C) This figure illustrates how the mean initial .04 vector shown in (A) will influence the precordial leads. In this case a Q wave will be recorded in Leads V-1, V-2, and V-3 and the initial .04 second of the QRS cycle will be resultantly zero in Leads V-4, V-5, and V-6. Although it is not illustrated, the ST segment would be elevated in Leads V-1, V-2, V-3, and isoelectric in Leads V-4, V-5, and V-6. The T waves would be inverted in Leads V-1, V-2, and V-3 and flat in Leads V-4, V-5, and V-6.

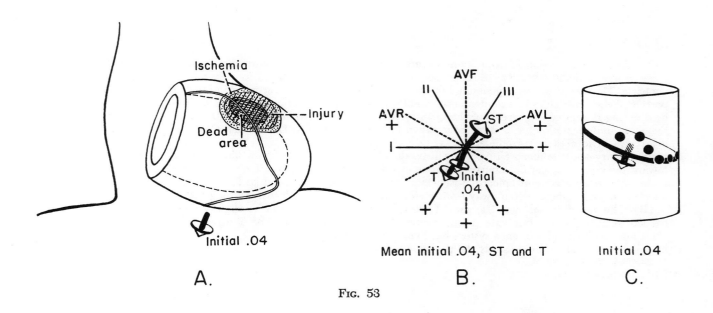

Ischemia

Injury

Dead area

Initial .04

A.

AVF

II   III

AVR   AVL
+   ST   +

I   +

T   Initial
.04
T

+   +
+

Mean initial .04, ST and T

B.

Initial .04

C.

Fig. 53

Fig. 54. (A) The myocardial infarction is located in the superior free wall and posterior basilar portion of the left ventricle. The electrical forces generated in the opposite portion of the ventricular muscle dominate the electrical field during the initial .04 second of the QRS cycle and the mean initial .04 vector is directed away from the dead area. The area is surrounded by a zone of epicardial injury and the mean ST vector will be directed toward the area of epicardial injury. The zone of injury is surrounded by a zone of epicardial ischemia and the mean T vector will be directed away from such an area.

(B) The mean initial .04, ST, and T vectors are treated as though they originate in the center of the chest and the hexaxial reference system has been superimposed. This enables one to study the projection of the vectors on the extremity lead axes. In this case a Q wave will be recorded in Leads I, aV_L, and aV_R and an R wave will be recorded in Leads II, III, and aV_F. The ST segment will be elevated in Leads I, aV_L, and aV_R and depressed in Leads II, III, and aV_F. The T wave will be inverted in Leads I and aV_L and upright in Leads II, III, aV_F, and aV_R.

(C) This figure illustrates how the mean initial .04 vector would influence the precordial leads in this particular case. Initial R waves will be recorded in all the precordial leads. Although it is not illustrated, the ST segment would be slightly depressed in all of the precordial leads. The T waves would be upright in all the precordial leads.

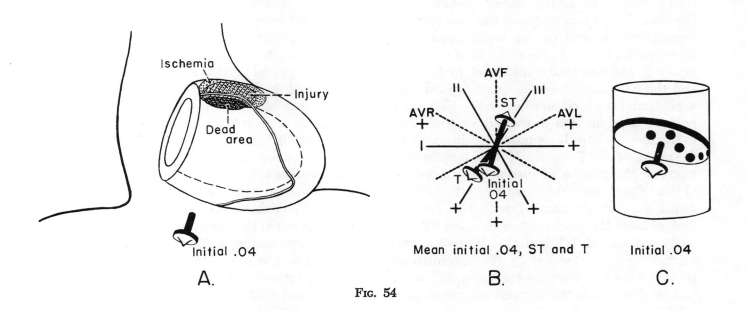

Ischemia

Injury

Dead area

Initial .04

A.

AVF

II

ST

III

AVR +

AVL +

I

+

T

Initial .04

+

+

+

Mean initial .04, ST and T

B.

Initial .04

C.

Fig. 54

(2) The Mean Spatial ST Vector. An abnormal ST segment displacement can be identified in the electrocardiograms of most patients with a recent myocardial infarction. The ST segment shift is due to an "injury current" produced by the zone of injury surrounding the area of myocardial necrosis and can be represented by a mean spatial vector. In the majority of cases the injury is predominantly epicardial in location and the ST vector tends to point toward that area. Under such circumstances the ST vector points toward an area of the left ventricle and is therefore relatively opposite in direction to the mean .04 and T vectors. If there is epicardial injury of the inferior or diaphragmatic surface of the left ventricle, the mean ST vector will be directed relatively parallel with the positive limb of Lead III, producing an elevated ST segment in Leads II, III, and aV$_F$. When the epicardial injury is located in the anterolateral region of the left ventricle the mean ST vector will be directed to the left and anteriorly, producing an elevated ST segment in Leads I, II, aV$_L$, and the left precordial leads. If the epicardial injury is located anteriorly, the mean ST vector will be directed anteriorly, producing an elevated ST segment in the right precordial leads.

At times the "injury current" will be located predominantly in the subendocardial region, under which circumstances the mean ST vector tends to point away from that area and as a rule is directed opposite to that of the mean QRS vector. If the vector representing subendocardial injury develops and persists for hours or days in a patient with a clinical picture of myocardial infarction, one should suspect subendocardial infarction. A transient ST vector of subendocardial injury is seen during angina pectoris.

There are many causes of ST segment displacement other than that associated with myocardial infarction. Some of the causes are mentioned briefly at this point but are enlarged on in other sections of the monograph. A prominent ST vector representing epicardial injury occurs in pericarditis and resembles the ST vector of myocardial infarction but tends to be parallel with the mean QRS vector. However, in pericarditis, no QRS abnormalities occur. The mean ST vector associated with digitalis medication is directed opposite to the mean QRS vector and therefore can closely resemble subendocardial injury. However, the mean T vector associated with digitalis medication is usually normally directed but is quite small and the QT interval is short. The ST vector occasionally seen in the normal subject, and the ST vector seen in left ventricular hypertrophy, right ventricular hypertrophy, left bundle branch block, and right bundle branch block are usually directed relatively parallel with the mean T vector which is quite unlike the ST-T vector relationship in myocardial infarction. A mean ST vector directed opposite to the mean QRS vector can be seen during angina pectoris, during tachycardia, as a result of the exercise tolerance test, following pulmonary embolism, or with anxiety and hyperventilation, and one must be cautious in making an etiologic electrocardiographic diagnosis without knowing all details of the clinical picture.

(3) **The Mean Spatial T Vector.** The ischemic myocardial cells surrounding the dead and injured zone produced by myocardial infarction are unable to repolarize in a normal manner. Because of this the mean T vector tends to be directed away from an area of ischemia located predominantly in the epicardial region of the heart.

In the normal adult the normal mean spatial T vector is usually located within 60° of the mean spatial QRS vector. It lies to the right of a markedly leftward mean spatial QRS vector and to the left of a vertical mean spatial QRS vector. It is always anterior to the mean spatial QRS vector and may be flush with the frontal plane or deviate 20° to 30° anteriorly or posteriorly from that plane. These are only general rules; certain exceptions are encountered and will be emphasized later.

When the T vector is directed away from an area of ischemia located in the left ventricle, the QRS-T angle may be more than 90°. If there is ischemia of the inferior or diaphragmatic surface of the left ventricle, the T vector will tend to rotate leftward to a point where the T waves will be inverted in Leads II, III, and aV$_F$. Under these circumstances the mean T vector is almost always located to the left of the mean QRS vector and the QRS-T angle may be abnormally wide. When the ischemia is anterolateral in location, the T vector is rotated to the right to a point where the T waves are inverted in Leads I and aV$_L$. Under these circumstances the mean T vector is located to the right of the mean QRS vector and the QRS-T angle may be abnormally wide. If the ischemia is located at the apex or involves the epicardial surface of the entire left ventricle, the T vector will point toward the right shoulder, causing the T waves to be inverted in Leads I, II, III, aV$_L$, and aV$_F$, producing a markedly abnormal QRS-T angle. If the ischemia involves the anterior portion of the left ventricle, the mean T vector may be directed abnormally posteriorly, causing the T waves at V-1, V-2, and V-3 to become negative.

Although the T vector changes listed above occur in myocardial infarction, similar changes may be seen in other pathological disorders and in totally benign physiological states. The reason for this is that many factors other than ischemia can influence the direction of the T vector. Since the T wave abnormalities of many different states, some serious and some unimportant, may be identical, one must depend on other electrocardiographic abnormalities and the clinical data in order to explain the T vector abnormality in a given case. For example, suppose the T vector is leftward and perpendicular to Lead III and is rotated 40° posteriorly, producing an inverted T wave in Leads V-1, V-2, and V-3. This type of abnormality may result from anterior ischemia of coronary occlusion but

can also be due to right ventricular ischemia associated with pulmonary embolism. On the other hand this type of finding may be entirely normal in children and young adults. Occasionally a T vector may be directed to the left, resembling diaphragmatic ischemia, in a variety of clinically unimportant physiologic states. Such a leftward T vector occurs in many normal subjects with standing, with increased heart rate from any cause, with head up tilting, during the Valsalva maneuver, after taking amyl nitrite or nitroglycerin, and from anxiety and hyperventilation. At times the T vector rotation is related to variations in the systolic size of the right ventricle, but frequently the exact cause of the apparent T abnormality is not known. When the heart rate is rapid, many individuals will develop a leftward deviated T vector and, surprisingly enough, a few susceptible persons will develop a leftward T with only slight increase in heart rate. From the preceding it can be seen that many electrocardiographic findings are similar and that in many instances the electrocardiogram is explained by knowledge of the clinical data and not vice versa.

Occasionally the ischemia associated with myocardial infarction is located principally in the subendocardial region. In such a case the T vector may become very large but retain a fairly normal position. This finding occurs early in the development of an infarction and usually gives way to the type of T vector change described above by the time the patient is first seen, but can, on occasion, last for several days.

In summary it can be stated that in classical myocardial infarction the mean spatial .04 vector and the mean spatial T vector will be directed away from the area of infarction and that the mean spatial ST vector will be directed toward the area of infarction. The .04 and T vectors may not be perfectly parallel with each other, and the ST vector may not be exactly 180° away from the .04 and T vectors. One reason for this is that the areas of dead, injured, and ischemic tissue may have dissimilar contours.

It is interesting to study the electrocardiograms of patients with multiple infarcts. Two abnormal .04 vectors, resulting from two separate myocardial infarcts, may produce a perfectly normally directed .04 vector since the recorded vector is the vector sum of the two abnormal vectors. Similarly, two abnormal ST vectors or two abnormal T vectors may produce normally directed ST or T vectors. The fact that two abnormal vectors can at times produce a normal vector should cause one to be cautious in assuming that changes toward the normal in serial electrocardiographic tracings always indicate improvement. In multiple infarcts the ST vector more accurately indicates the area of most recent infarct since previous injury effects subside faster than ischemic or dead effects.

The abnormal vectors seen in myocardial infarction vary with the age of the infarction. As the infarct heals, the ST vector disappears first, usually in two to three weeks. Occasionally after several weeks or months the abnormal T vector may return to normal and on rare occasions the dead zone vector may become smaller and finally vanish.

The electrocardiograms shown in fig. 55 through 70 illustrate the vector abnormalities of myocardial infarction occurring in various portions of the left ventricle. The recognition of a myocardial infarction is much more important than the localization of a myocardial infarct, and therefore one should not be misled by the attempts at localization in this monograph and in the literature. In reality it is sufficient to report an electrocardiogram as indicating a myocardial infarction and not specify its location.

119

FIG. 55. The electrocardiogram of a patient, 55 years of age, showing an acute posteroinferior myocardial infarction with lateral involvement.

(A) The frontal plane projection of the mean QRS, ST, T, and initial .04 vectors are shown. The frontal plane projection of the spatial QRS loop is also shown. Note that the QRS complex is equiphasic in Lead II and can be represented by a mean vector directed perpendicular to Lead II. The T wave is smallest in Lead III and can be represented by a mean vector directed perpendicular to Lead III. The ST segment is markedly elevated in Lead II, slightly depressed in Lead aV_L. This ST segment displacement can be represented by a mean vector directed just to the right of the positive limb of Lead II. The initial .04 second of the QRS loop is resultantly negative in Lead III and aV_F and is positive in Lead aV_R. A mean vector representing the forces generated during the initial .04 second of the QRS cycle will be directed just to the right of the negative limb of Lead III. The QRS loop travels in a clockwise manner.

(B) The spatial QRS loop is shown. The initial portion of the loop, represented by the first vector, is directed slightly to the right and anteriorly; the second portion of the loop, represented by the second vector, is directed slightly to the left and anteriorly; and the third portion of the loop, represented by the third vector, is directed to the left and is flush with the frontal plane. The subsequent portions of the loop are directed to the left and posteriorly.

(C) The mean ST vector is rotated approximately 30° posteriorly because the transitional ST pathway passes between electrode positions V-3 and V-4.

(D) The mean T vector is rotated approximately 30° anteriorly because all of the precordial leads record tall, upright T waves.

(E) Final summary figure showing the spatial arrangement of the vectors. The mean spatial initial .04 vector is located abnormally to the left of the horizontally directed mean QRS vector and indicates an inferior dead zone. The mean ST vector is directed downward, to the left, and slightly posteriorly toward the area of inferior and lateral epicardial injury. The mean T vector is in a normal position but has tremendous magnitude. This indicates generalized subendocardial ischemia. This finding occurs transiently at the onset of myocardial infarction; later the mean T vector will be directed away from the area of epicardial ischemia surrounding the infarct.

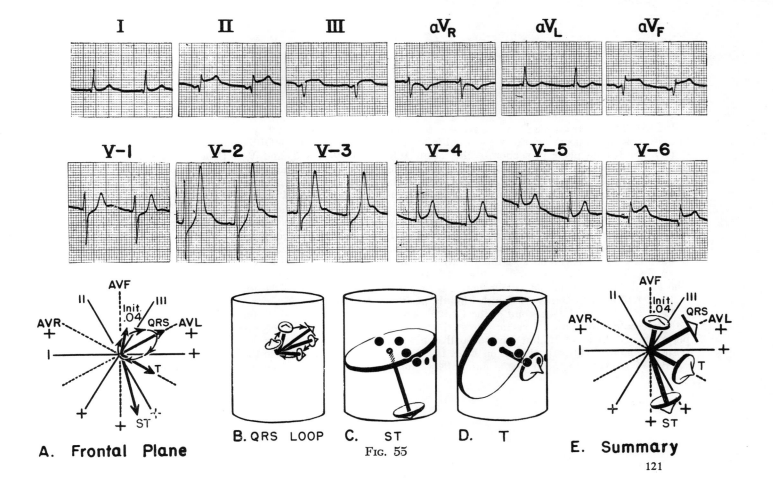

I II III aV_R aV_L aV_F

V-1 V-2 V-3 V-4 V-5 V-6

A. Frontal Plane

B. QRS LOOP

C. ST

D. T

E. Summary

FIG. 55

121

Fig. 56. The electrocardiogram of a patient, 62 years of age, showing an acute inferior myocardial infarction.

(A) The frontal plane projection of the mean QRS, ST, T, and initial .04 vectors. The mean QRS vector is directed perpendicular to Lead aV_F because the QRS complex is resultantly zero in Lead aV_F. The ST segment displacement is greatest in Lead III and least in Lead aV_R and can be represented by a mean vector directed parallel with the positive limb of Lead III. The mean T vector is directed just to the left of the positive limb of Lead aV_F because the T wave is slightly positive in Lead I and large and positive in Lead aV_F. The initial .04 second of the QRS complex is negative in Lead III and aV_F and is resultantly slightly positive in Lead II. The initial .04 second of the QRS cycle can be represented by a mean vector directed relatively perpendicular to Lead II, but located so that a small positive quantity will be projected on Lead II.

(B), (C), (D) The mean spatial initial .04 vector is rotated approximately 80° anteriorly because the initial .04 second of the QRS complex is resultantly positive in V-1, V-2, V-3, and V-4. (The Q wave in V-5 is .02 second in duration and the transitional pathway for the initial .04 vector lies near V-6.) The mean spatial ST vector is rotated posteriorly since the ST segment is depressed in all the precordial leads. The mean spatial T vector is tilted at least 15° anteriorly since all the precordial leads record upright T waves.

(E) The mean spatial initial .04 vector is abnormal in position because it is located too far to the left of the horizontally directed mean spatial QRS vector. The mean spatial ST vector is directed toward the area of inferior and posterior epicardial injury and the mean spatial initial .04 vector is directed away from the area of posterior myocardial necrosis. The infarction is clinically only three hours old and the mean T vector has not yet assumed the position of being directed away from the ischemia surrounding an area of necrosis.

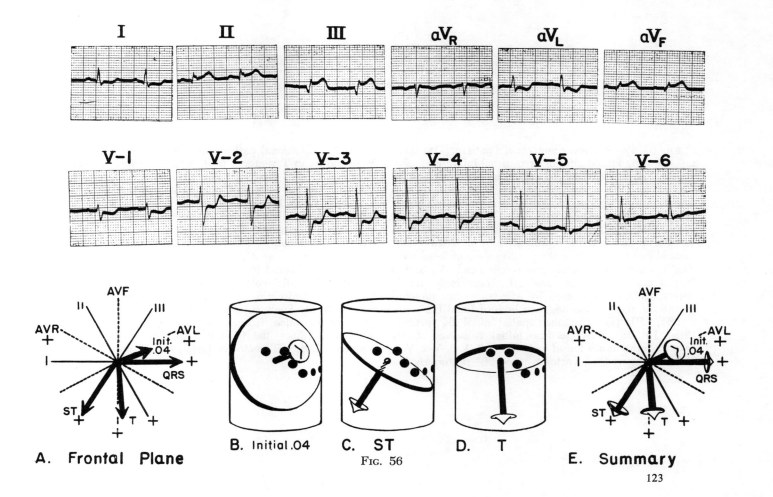

I II III aV_R aV_L aV_F

V-1 V-2 V-3 V-4 V-5 V-6

A. Frontal Plane

B. Initial .04

C. ST

D. T

E. Summary

Fig. 56

123

Fig. 57. The electrocardiogram of a patient, 50 years of age, showing an old inferior myocardial infarction.

(A) The mean initial .04 vector is resultantly zero in Lead II and is therefore perpendicular to Lead II. It is drawn in the direction indicated because deep Q waves are present in Leads III and aV_F. The QRS complex is largest and positive in Lead I and slightly negative in Lead aV_F and can be represented by a mean vector located just to the left of the positive limb of Lead aV_F. The T wave is just barely positive in Lead aV_R and is largest and negative in Lead III. Accordingly, the T waves can be represented by a mean vector directed just to the right of the negative limb of Lead III.

(B), (C), (D) The mean spatial initial .04 vector is tilted 10° anteriorly because initial R waves of .04 second duration are found in Leads V-2, V-3, V-4, V-5, V-6. The mean QRS vector is tilted 20° posteriorly be-cause the transitional pathway passes between V-2 and V-3. The mean T vector is flush with the frontal plane. Note how the T waves are low and upright in Leads V-1 and V-4 but large and upright in Leads V-2, V-3, V-5, V-6. When the mean T vector is located as indicated, it is possible for the electrodes located in the V-1 *and* V-4 positions to record near the transitional pathway produced by the T wave.

(E) The mean spatial initial .04 and T vectors are abnormally directed to the left of the horizontally directed mean QRS vector. These vectors are directed away from the inferior or diaphragmatic surface of the left ventricle. Such an infarction, sometimes called a posterior infarction, is more properly called an inferior infarction. (Since the infarction in this case is four months old, the ST vector is quite small.)

124

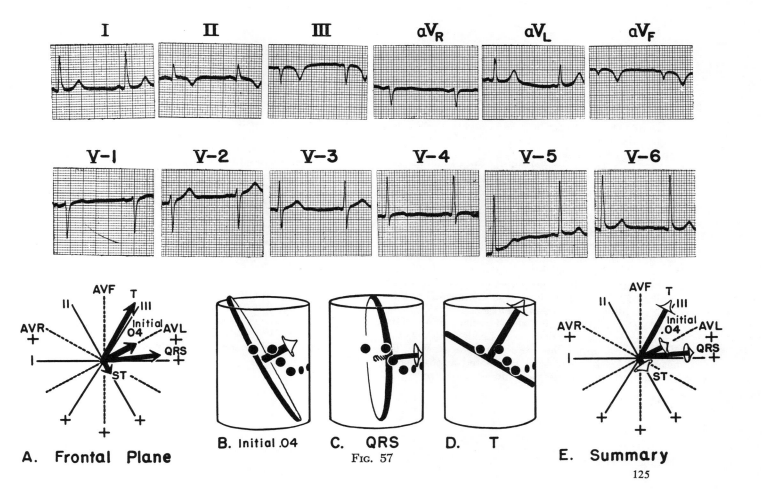

I II III aV_R aV_L aV_F

V-1 V-2 V-3 V-4 V-5 V-6

A. Frontal Plane

B. Initial .04

C. QRS

D. T

E. Summary

Fig. 57

125

FIG. 58. The electrocardiogram of a patient, 49 years of age, showing an old inferior myocardial infarction with only QRS changes.

(A) The first .04 second of the QRS complexes is positive in Lead I and negative in Lead II and largest and negative in Lead III. This QRS abnormality can be represented by a mean vector directed relatively perpendicular to Lead II. The mean QRS vector is slightly negative in Lead aV_L and slightly positive in Lead I and can be represented by a vector located slightly to the right of the positive limb of Lead II. The T wave is largest in Lead I and slightly positive in Lead aV_F and can be represented by a mean vector directed relatively parallel with Lead I but directed so that a small positive quantity will be projected on Lead aV_F.

(B), (C), (D) The initial .04 second of the QRS complexes is large and positive in Leads V-1, V-2, V-3, V-4, V-5 and approaches resultant zero at V-6. The mean initial .04 vector must be rotated approximately 75° anteriorly to produce such findings in the precordial leads. The mean spatial QRS vector is rotated 20° posteriorly because the transitional pathway passes through electrode position V-3. The mean spatial T vector is rotated 15° anteriorly because all the precordial T waves are upright, V-1 being the smallest.

(E) The mean spatial initial .04 vector is directed to the left of a vertically directed mean QRS vector. The spatial QRS-T angle is approximately 65°. The only definite abnormality is that of the position of the mean initial .04 vector. This patient had a clinical history and electrocardiographic evidence of a posterior myocardial infarction 15 years prior to the above tracing. At times it is extremely difficult to determine when an old inferior infarction is present. If the .04 vector is located far enough to the left to produce a Q wave in Leads II, III, and aV_F—the latter of .04 second duration —and the mean QRS vector is in a vertical position, then inferior myocardial infarction is likely. [See QRS loop in 70 (A).]

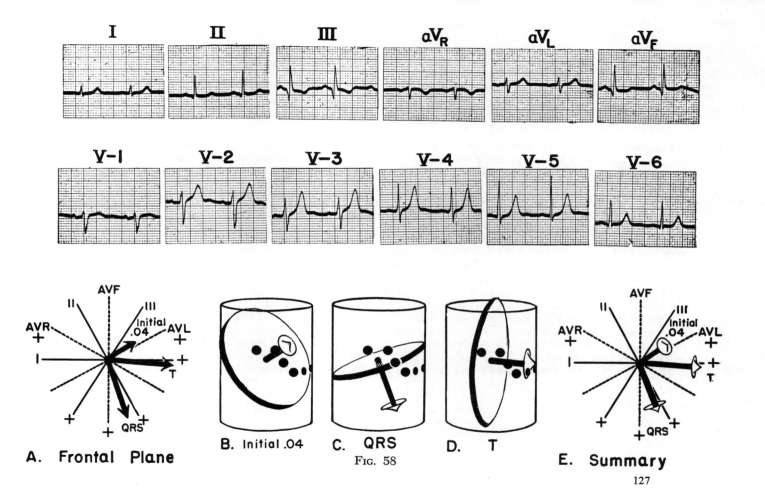

I II III aV_R aV_L aV_F

V-1 V-2 V-3 V-4 V-5 V-6

A. Frontal Plane

B. Initial .04

C. QRS

D. T

Fig. 58

E. Summary

127

Fig. 59. The electrocardiogram of a patient, 34 years of age, showing an old inferior myocardial infarction.

(A) The frontal plane projection of the mean QRS, T, and initial .04 vectors. The initial .04 second of the QRS complex is resultantly negative in Leads III and aV$_F$ and resultantly slightly negative in Lead II and resultantly slightly positive in Lead aV$_R$. These initial forces can be represented by a mean vector directed relatively parallel with Lead III but located so that a small positive quantity will be projected on Lead aV$_R$. The QRS complex is resultantly zero in Lead III and can be represented by a vector perpendicular to Lead III. The T waves are large and negative in Leads II and III and slightly positive in Lead I. Such T waves can be represented by a mean vector directed relatively parallel with the negative limb of Lead aV$_F$ but located so that a small positive quantity will be projected on Lead I.

(B), (C), (D) The mean spatial initial .04 vector is directed approximately 15° anteriorly because V-1, V-2, V-3 are resultantly positive during the first .04 second of the QRS cycle and Leads V-4, V-5, V-6 record from the transitional pathway for they are negative during the first .02 second and positive during the next .02 second. The mean QRS vector is flush with the frontal plane since V-1 records a resultantly negative deflection and V-2 records a resultantly positive deflection. The mean spatial T vector is rotated 5° posteriorly since the T waves are upright in V-1 and V-2 and negative in V-3, V-4, V-5, and V-6.

(E) The mean spatial initial .04 and T vectors are directed abnormally to the left of the mean spatial QRS vector. The QRS-T angle is approximately 115°. The .04 and T vectors are directed away from the inferior and posterior surface of the left ventricle. The magnitude of the QRS complex in V-3 is suggestive but not diagnostic of left ventricular hypertrophy.

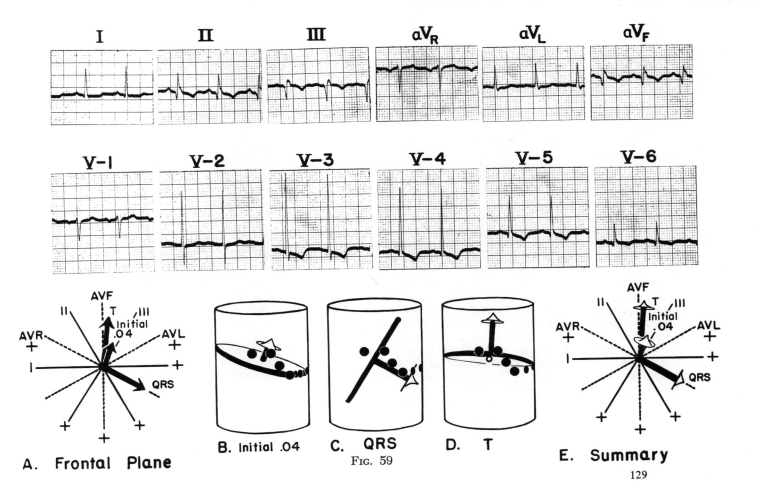

I   II   III   aV_R   aV_L   aV_F

V-1   V-2   V-3   V-4   V-5   V-6

A. Frontal Plane

B. Initial .04

C. QRS

D. T

E. Summary

Fig. 59

129

Fig. 60. The electrocardiogram of a patient, 53 years of age, recorded 11 days after an acute inferior infarction.

(A) The QRS complex is largest and negative in Lead III and resultantly zero in Lead aV_R. QRS complexes with these characteristics can be represented by a mean vector parallel to the negative limb of Lead III. The first .04 second of the QRS complex is deeply negative in Lead III and slightly negative in Lead II and can be represented by a mean vector directed relatively parallel with the positive limb of Lead aV_L but directed so that a small negative quantity will be projected on Lead II. The T waves are deeply inverted in Leads II, III, aV_F and slightly positive in Lead I. Such T waves can be represented by a mean vector directed relatively parallel with the negative limb of Lead aV_F but directed so that a small positive quantity will be projected on Lead I. The ST segment is slightly elevated in Leads II and III and isoelectric in Lead I and can be represented by a mean vector directed perpendicular to Lead I.

(B), (C), (D) The mean initial .04 spatial vector is approximately flush with the frontal plane because the initial forces are negative in Lead V-1 and positive in Leads V-2, V-3, V-4, V-5, V-6. The mean spatial ST vector is rotated at least 15° anteriorly because the ST segment is slightly elevated in all the precordial leads. The mean T vector is rotated about 5° posteriorly because the T waves are positive in Leads V-1 and V-2 and negative in Leads V-3, V-4, V-5, V-6.

(E) Final summary figure illustrating the spatial arrangements of the vectors. The mean initial .04 vector has a normal relationship with the mean QRS vector but the irregularity of the initial portion of the QRS loop is suggestive of infarction. (Note notching of initial .04 portion of QRS in Lead II.) In this case many of the diaphragmatic QRS forces have been destroyed, thereby altering the mean QRS so that marked left axis deviation results. The mean T vector is located abnormally to the left of the mean QRS vector and is directed away from the inferior, anterior, and apical surfaces of the left ventricle. Note that the QRS-T angle is only 25°. The inverted T waves in Leads V-4, V-5, V-6 are interesting and it should be pointed out that a large zone of anterolateral ischemia surrounding a single infarction can produce such a finding and that one need not postulate two infarctions. The mean spatial ST vector is directed toward an area of inferior and anterior injury.

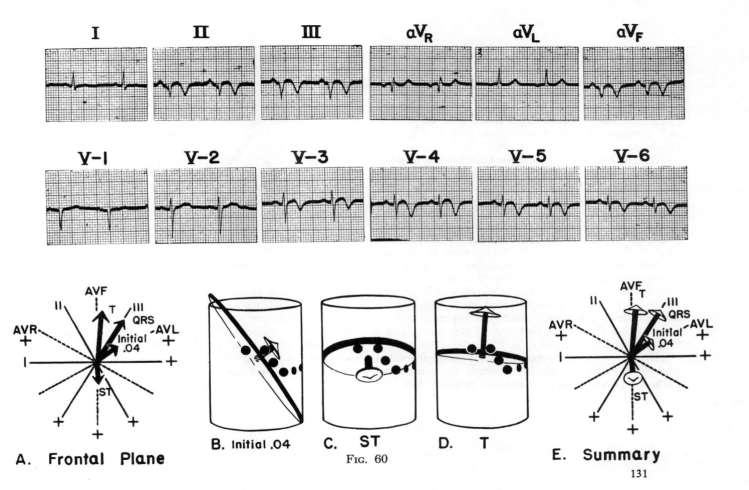

I II III aV_R aV_L aV_F

V-1 V-2 V-3 V-4 V-5 V-6

A. Frontal Plane B. Initial .04 C. ST D. T E. Summary

Fig. 60

131

FIG. 61. The electrocardiogram of a patient, 74 years old, showing an anteroseptal dead zone and inferior ischemia.

(A) The first .04 second of the QRS cycle is negative in Lead III and isoelectric in Lead aV_F. The forces generated during the initial .04 second of the QRS cycle can be represented by a mean vector directed perpendicular to Lead aV_F and directed toward the positive pole of Lead I. The QRS complex is largest in Lead I and slightly negative in Lead III and positive in Lead aV_F. Such complexes can be represented by a mean vector located between a perpendicular to Lead III and a perpendicular to Lead aV_F. The T wave is large and negative in Lead III and slightly negative in Lead aV_R. Such T waves can be represented by a mean vector directed relatively parallel with the negative limb of Lead III but directed so that a small negative quantity will be projected on Lead aV_R.

(B), (C), (D) The mean initial .04 vector is rotated posteriorly approximately 30° because the transitional pathway passes through electrode position V-3. (It should be noted that the R wave is absent in V-1 and V-2. There is a Q wave of .02 second duration in V-3 and an R wave for the second .02 second in Lead V-3. This indicates that the first .02 second forces are directed more posteriorly than the next .02 second forces. This finding is characteristic of anteroseptal dead zone.) The mean QRS vector must be rotated 40° posteriorly because the transitional pathway passes between V-3 and V-4. The mean T vector is rotated an unknown number of degrees anteriorly since all precordial T deflections are upright.

(E) The mean spatial initial .04 vector is directed in a normal manner when viewed in the frontal plane. The initial forces are abnormal when viewed in space because the initial .02 second forces are directed more posteriorly than the next .02 second forces indicating anteroseptal dead zone. The mean T vector is rotated abnormally to the left and anteriorly and is directed away from an area of posterior and inferior myocardial ischemia. [See QRS loop in fig. 70 (B).]

132

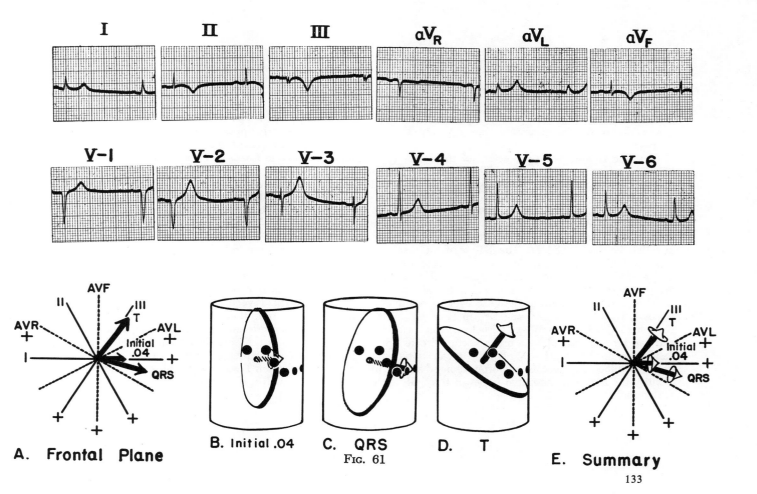

I   II   III   aV_R   aV_L   aV_F

V-1   V-2   V-3   V-4   V-5   V-6

A. Frontal Plane

B. Initial .04   C. QRS   D. T

FIG. 61

E. Summary

133

FIG. 62. The electrocardiogram of a patient, 71 years of age, with myocardial infarction showing only T wave changes.

(A) The frontal plane projection of the mean QRS, ST, T, and initial .04 vectors. The QRS complex is resultantly zero in Lead III and positive in Leads I and II. Accordingly, the mean QRS vector is directed perpendicular to Lead III. The T wave is isoelectric in Lead aV_L and negative in Lead II and III and can be represented by a mean vector directed parallel with the negative limb of Lead II. The ST segment displacement is slight but is greatest and negative in Lead II and least in Lead aV_L and can be represented by a mean vector directed parallel with the negative limb of Lead II. The initial .04 second of the QRS cycle is positive in Leads I, II, aV_L, aV_F, and negative in Lead aV_R. This portion of the QRS complex is isoelectric in Lead III and can be represented by a mean vector directed perpendicular to Lead III. (When the mean initial .04 vector is difficult to plot, one is often obliged simply to identify the fact that the initial forces of the QRS cycle are normally directed.)

(B), (C), (D) The mean spatial initial .04 vector is rotated posteriorly approximately 20° because the transitional pathway passes through V-3. There is a small initial R wave in Leads V-1 and V-2 of .01 to .02 duration but the resultant of the forces during the first .04 second is negative in Leads V-1 and V-2. The mean ST vector is rotated approximately 20° anteriorly since the ST segment is slightly elevated in V-1, V-2 and depressed in V-4, V-5, V-6. The mean T vector is rotated approximately 10° posteriorly because the T wave is flat in V-1 and negative in V-2, V-3, V-4, V-5, V-6.

(E) Final summary figure illustrating the spatial arrangement of the vectors. The principal abnormality is that of the direction of the T vector. The QRS-T angle is 150° and the T vector is quite large. The T vector is directed away from the apical region of the left ventricle and probably represents severe ischemia of that region. Although this is the only definite abnormality, one can usually be certain that a certain amount of cell death has occurred when T waves with this magnitude are seen in a patient with a clinical story compatible with coronary occlusion.

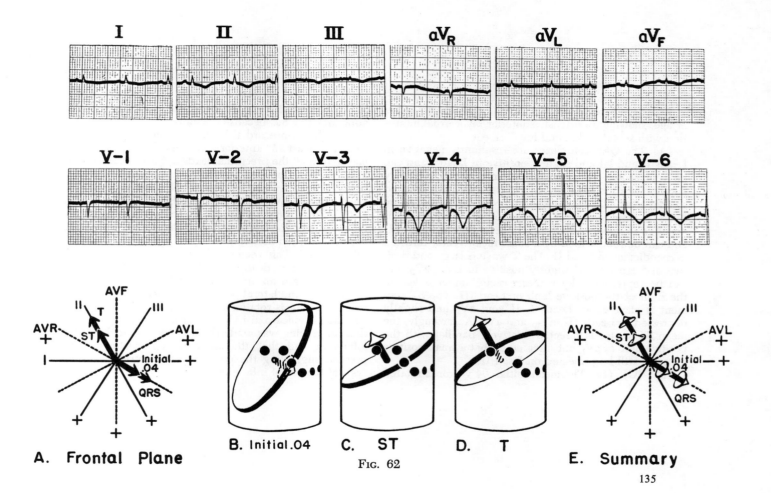

I II III aV_R aV_L aV_F

V-1 V-2 V-3 V-4 V-5 V-6

A. Frontal Plane

B. Initial .04   C. ST   D. T

E. Summary

Fig. 62

135

Fig. 63. The electrocardiogram of a patient, 48 years of age, showing an extensive anterior myocardial infarction with septal and lateral involvement.

(A) The QRS complexes are resultantly negative in Leads II and III and slightly positive in Lead I and can be represented by a mean vector directed relatively parallel with the negative limb of Lead aV_F but directed so that a small positive quantity will be projected on Lead I. The initial .04 portion of the QRS cycle is negative in Leads I and aV_L and positive in Lead III and can be represented by a small mean vector directed perpendicular to Lead II. The T wave is large and positive in Lead III and slightly positive in Lead aV_R and can be represented by a mean vector directed just to the right of the positive limb of Lead III. The ST segment is elevated in Leads I, II, and aV_L and slightly depressed in Leads III, aV_R, and aV_F. Accordingly, the mean ST vector is directed relatively parallel with the positive limb of aV_L but directed so that a small positive quantity will be projected on Lead II.

(B), (C), (D) The mean initial .04 vector is rotated markedly posterior and deviated from the frontal plane approximately 80° because the initial .04 second is negative in all the precordial leads. The mean ST vector is rotated at least 45° anteriorly because the ST segment is elevated in all the precordial leads but is less elevated in V-1 and V-6. The mean T vector is approximately flush with the frontal plane because the T wave is upright in Lead V-1 and inverted in Leads V-2, V-3, V-4, V-5, V-6.

(E) Final summary figure illustrating the spatial arrangement of the vectors. The mean spatial initial .04 vector is located abnormally to the right and is posteriorly directed. This vector is directed away from a large area of anterior dead zone. The mean ST vector is directed toward an area of epicardial injury located in the anterior and lateral portion of the left ventricle. The mean T vector is rotated away from an area of anterior and lateral epicardial ischemia. It is interesting to note that the tracing was made three months after the acute infarction and that the abnormal ST vector is still present, suggesting the possibility of ventricular aneurysm at the site of infarction.

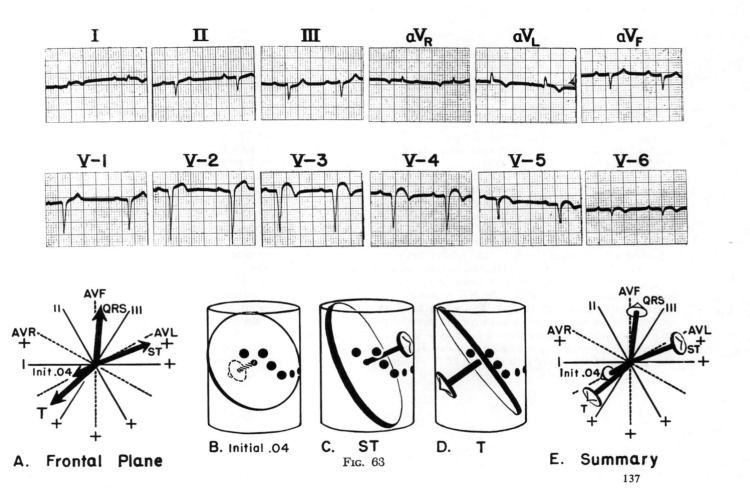

I II III aV$_R$ aV$_L$ aV$_F$

V-1 V-2 V-3 V-4 V-5 V-6

A. Frontal Plane

B. Initial .04

C. ST

D. T

Fig. 63

E. Summary

137

FIG. 64. The electrocardiogram of a patient, 56 years of age, showing a large anteroseptal and lateral myocardial infarction.

(A) The QRS complex is large and negative in Lead II and resultantly slightly positive in Lead aV_R. QRS complexes with these characteristics can be represented by a mean QRS vector directed relatively parallel with the negative limb of Lead III but directed so that a small positive quantity will be projected on Lead aV_R. The first .04 second of the QRS loop is resultantly zero in Lead aV_R, positive in Lead III, and negative in Lead aV_L and can be represented by a mean vector directed perpendicular to Lead aV_R. The ST segment is depressed in Leads I and II and elevated in Lead aV_R and can be represented by a mean vector directed just to the right of the negative limb of Lead aV_F. The mean T vector is directed perpendicular to Lead II because the T wave is resultantly zero in Lead II.

(B), (C), (D) The mean spatial initial .04 vector is rotated 80° posteriorly because the initial .04 second of the QRS complex is negative in V-1, V-2, V-3, V-4, and V-5, and is resultantly zero in V-6. The mean ST vector is rotated approximately 20° anteriorly because the ST segment is elevated in V-1, V-2, V-3, and is depressed in V-4, V-5, V-6. The mean T vector is flush with the frontal plane because the transitional pathway passes between V-1 and V-2.

(E) Final summary figure illustrating the spatial arrangement of the vectors. The mean initial .04 vector is directed abnormally posteriorly. It is directed away from the anterior surface of the left ventricle. The mean T vector is located abnormally to the right and is directed away from an extensive area of anterolateral ischemia.

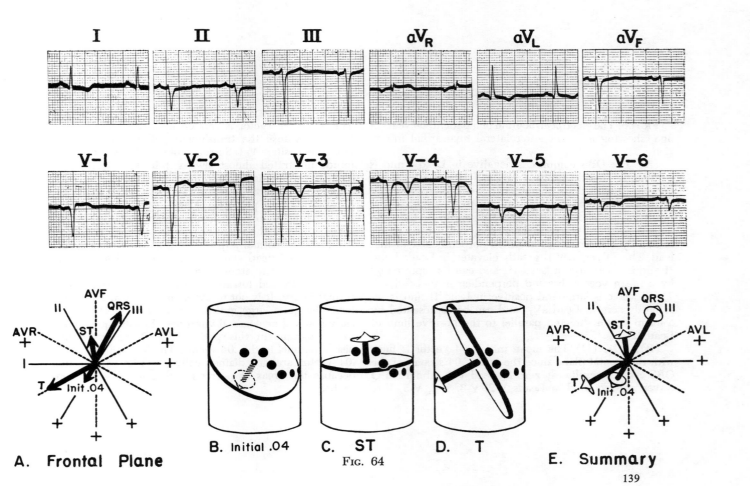

I II III aV$_R$ aV$_L$ aV$_F$

V-1 V-2 V-3 V-4 V-5 V-6

A. Frontal Plane

B. Initial .04

C. ST

D. T

E. Summary

Fig. 64

139

Fig. 65. The electrocardiogram of a patient, 59 years of age, showing a recent anterolateral myocardial infarction.

(A) The QRS complex is negative in Lead I and is resultantly slightly positive in Lead II and aV_R. QRS complexes with these characteristics can be represented by a mean vector directed slightly to the right of the positive limb of Lead III. The .04 second of the QRS loop is resultantly zero in Lead aV_R and can be represented by a mean vector directed perpendicular to that lead. The ST segment is greatly elevated in Leads I and II and is isoelectric in Lead III and can be represented by a mean vector directed perpendicular to Lead III. The T wave is large and positive in Lead II and is resultantly zero in Lead aV_L, and can be represented by a mean vector directed parallel to the positive limb of Lead II.

(B), (C), (D) The mean initial .04 vector is flush with the frontal plane since the initial .04 second of the QRS cycle is resultantly zero in Lead V-1. Abnormal Q waves are recorded in Leads V-2, V-3, V-4, V-5, V-6.

The mean ST vector is rotated approximately 10° anteriorly because the transitional pathway passes near electrode position V-1. ST segment elevations of the magnitude illustrated almost always indicate epicardial injury of myocardial infarction. The mean T vector is rotated 15° or more anteriorly because the T waves are upright in all the precordial leads.

(E) Final summary figure illustrating the spatial arrangement of the vectors. The mean initial .04 vector is directed abnormally to the right as is the entire QRS loop. The .04 dead zone vector is directed away from an area of anterolateral myocardial necrosis. The ST vector is directed toward an area of anterolateral epicardial injury. It is not uncommon for the mean T vector to be quite large and normally directed during the early hours of myocardial infarction. In subsequent electrocardiograms in this patient the T vector became nearly parallel to the .04 vector. The ST vector and the .04 vector are not diametrically opposite in direction because the areas of necrosis and injury are not concentric.

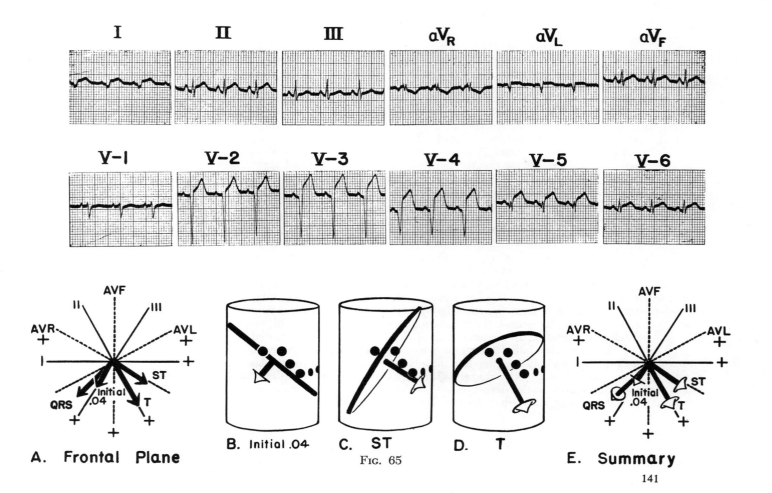

A. Frontal Plane

B. Initial .04

C. ST

D. T

E. Summary

Fig. 65

141

Fig. 66. The electrocardiogram of a patient, 58 years of age, showing an extensive anterolateral and septal myocardial infarction.

(A) The QRS complex is positive in Lead III and resultantly slightly positive in Lead II and resultantly zero in Lead aV_R and can be represented by a vector directed parallel with Lead III. The initial .04 second of the QRS cycle is positive in Leads II, III, and aV_F and negative in Leads aV_R and aV_L and resultantly zero in Lead I. Accordingly, the mean initial .04 vector is directed perpendicular to Lead I. The ST segment displacement is positive in Leads I and aV_L and negative in Leads III and aV_F and slightly negative in Lead II and can be represented by a mean vector located between the positive limb of Lead aV_L and the negative limb of Lead III. The T wave is large and negative in Lead I, slightly negative in Lead II, and slightly positive in Lead aV_F and can be represented by a mean vector located just to the right of the negative limb of aV_L.

(B), (C), (D) The mean initial .04 vector is rotated approximately 35° posteriorly because the transitional pathway passes through V-4. (Note that the QRS duration appears to be shorter in the deflection at V-4 than it is at V-3 and V-5, suggesting that the initial portion of V-4 deflection is almost isoelectric which means that the vectors are perpendicular to the axis of this lead during this interval.) The mean ST vector is rotated approximately 80° anteriorly since all the precordial deflections have elevated ST segments. The mean T vector is rotated approximately 10° anteriorly since the T wave is upright in V-1 and V-2, and isoelectric in V-3 and inverted in V-4, V-5, and V-6.

(E) Final summary figure illustrating the spatial arrangement of the vectors. The mean initial .04 vector is directed abnormally posteriorly and points away from the anteroseptal region of the left ventricle. The ST vector is directed toward the anterior region of epicardial injury. The mean T vector is directed away from an area of anterolateral ischemia. It is interesting to note that myocardial infarction can superficially resemble right ventricular hypertrophy. In this case there is right axis deviation and there is a deep S wave in V-5 and V-6. The mean initial .04 and mean QRS vectors are directed posteriorly in this case rather than anteriorly as in right ventricular hypertrophy. A large abnormal ST vector having the direction shown above is not seen in right ventricular hypertrophy. [See QRS loop in fig. 70 (C).]

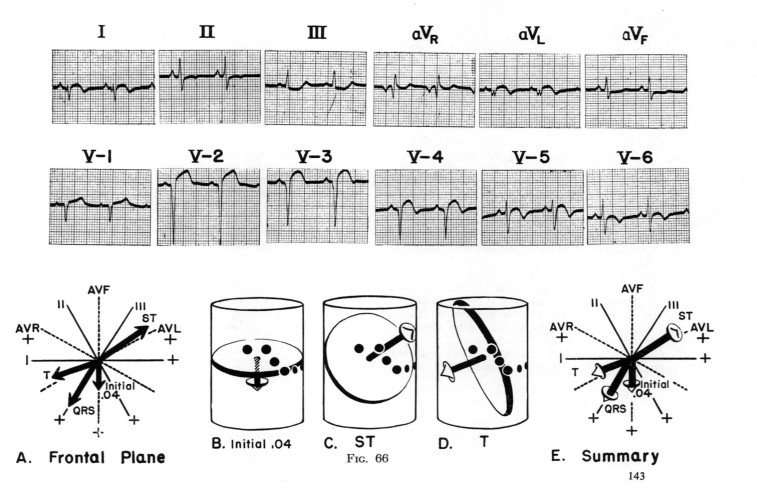

I II III aV_R aV_L aV_F

V-1 V-2 V-3 V-4 V-5 V-6

A. Frontal Plane

B. Initial .04

C. ST

D. T

E. Summary

Fig. 66

143

FIG. 67. The electrocardiogram of a patient, 65 years of age, showing an acute anteroseptal myocardial infarction.

(A) The mean QRS vector is perpendicular to Lead III because the QRS complex is resultantly zero in Lead III. The initial .04 second of the QRS cycle is negative in Leads I and aV_L and positive in Leads III and aV_F and resultantly zero in Lead II and can be represented by a mean vector directed perpendicular to Lead II. The ST segment displacement is greatest and positive in Leads I and II while there is little displacement in Lead III. Accordingly, the mean ST vector is directed perpendicular to Lead III. The T wave is large and positive in Lead II and slightly negative in Lead aV_L and can be represented by a mean vector directed just to the right of the positive limb of Lead II.

(B), (C), (D) The mean initial .04 vector is rotated approximately 80° posteriorly because there are initial negative deflections in Leads V-1, V-2, V-3, V-4, V-5 and an initial positive deflection in Lead V-6. The mean ST vector is rotated approximately 80° anteriorly because all precordial ST segment deflections are markedly elevated. The mean T vector is rotated at least 15° anteriorly since the T waves are upright in all the precordial leads.

(E) Final summary figure illustrating the spatial arrangement of the vectors. The mean initial .04 vector is directed abnormally posteriorly and is pointed away from an anteroseptal region of the left ventricle. The mean ST vector is abnormally prominent and is directed toward an area of anterior epicardial injury. The T vector is located in a fairly normal position because this is a very early tracing. Later electrocardiograms show the mean T vector directed away from the anterior surface of the heart.

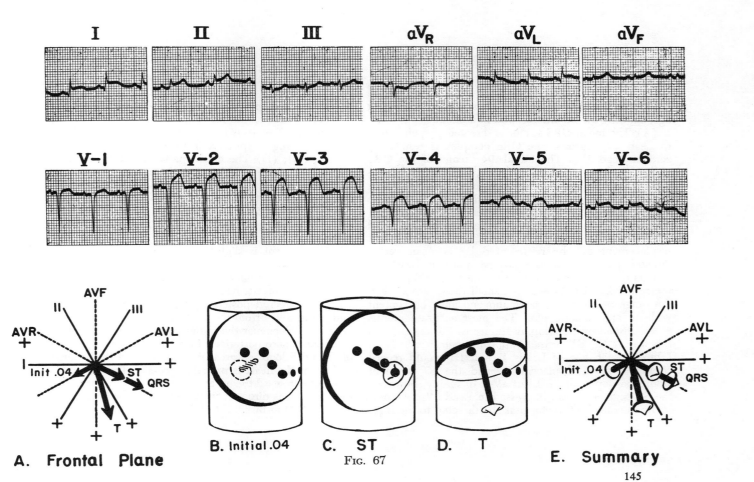

I II III aV_R aV_L aV_F

V-1 V-2 V-3 V-4 V-5 V-6

A. Frontal Plane

B. Initial .04

C. ST

D. T

E. Summary

Fig. 67

Fig. 68. The electrocardiogram of a patient, 62 years of age, showing an old anteroseptal infarction.

(A) The mean QRS vector is directed perpendicular to Lead aV_F because the QRS complex is resultantly zero in Lead aV_F. The initial .04 second of the QRS cycle is positive in Leads I, II, aV_L, and aV_F and negative in Lead III and can be represented by a mean vector directed between the negative limb of aV_R and the positive limb of Lead I. There is very little ST segment displacement but this interval appears elevated in Lead III and slightly elevated in Lead II. The ST segment displacement can be represented by a mean vector directed parallel with the positive limb of Lead III. (Actually, in such a case the ST segment should be depressed in Lead I. When such small forces are studied the range of error is greater and one must be content with an approximate plot. The most accurate plot is accomplished by studying all the leads. For instance, in this tracing the ST segment appears isoelectric in Lead I but in such a case Leads II and III would record equally positive displacements and the ST segment would be depressed in Lead aV_R. In reality, however, the ST segment is not depressed in Lead aV_R. Accordingly, the mean ST vector must be directed to the right

of the positive limb of Lead aV_F.) The mean T vector is directed just to the left of the positive limb of aV_F because the T wave is upright in Leads II, III, and aV_F but is only slightly positive in Lead I.

(B), (C), (D) The mean spatial initial .04 vector is rotated 30° posteriorly because there is an initial negative deflection in V-1, V-2, V-3 and an initial positive deflection of the QRS in V-4, V-5, V-6. The mean QRS vector is rotated 20° posteriorly because the transitional pathway passes between V-2 and V-3. The mean ST vector is small and is rotated about 80° anteriorly because the ST segment is slightly elevated in V-1, V-2, V-3, V-4, V-5.

(E) Final summary figure illustrating the spatial arrangement of the vectors. Note that the initial .04 vector is directed posteriorly to the mean QRS vector and points away from the anteroseptal region of the left ventricle. Whenever the initial portion of the QRS loop is directed more posteriorly than the subsequent portion of the QRS loop, an area of dead zone on the anterior surface of the heart is probably present. The ST vector is directed toward the anterior surface of the heart while the T vector is directed away from the anterior surface. [See QRS loop in fig. 70 (D).]

146

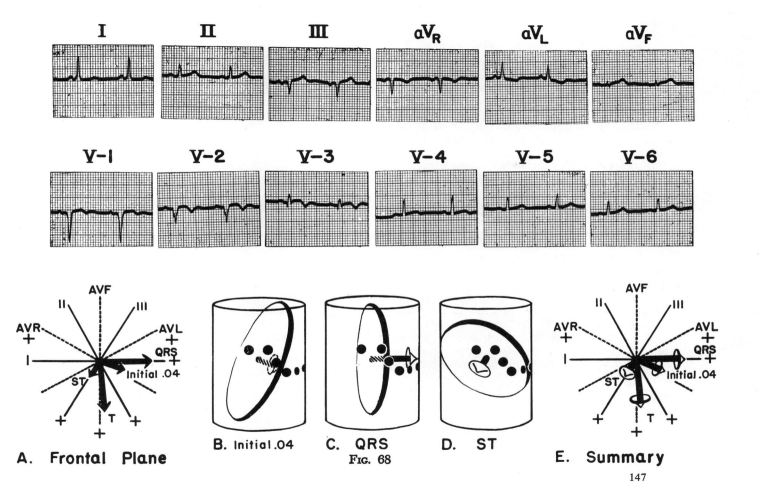

I   II   III   aV$_R$ aV$_L$ aV$_F$

V-1   V-2   V-3   V-4   V-5   V-6

A. Frontal Plane

B. Initial .04

C. QRS

D. ST

E. Summary

FIG. 68

147

Fig. 69. The electrocardiogram of a patient, 70 years of age, showing an anteroseptal and inferior myocardial infarction.

(A) The mean QRS vector is directed parallel with the negative limb of Lead III because the QRS complex is large and negative in Lead III and resultantly zero in Lead aV_R. The initial .04 second of the QRS complex is negative in Leads III and aV_F and appears isoelectric in Lead II and negative in Lead aV_R. Accordingly, the mean initial .04 vector is directed perpendicular to Lead II. The mean ST vector is almost perpendicular to Lead I and is extremely small when viewed in the frontal plane. The mean T vector is perpendicular to Lead I because the T wave is isoelectric in that lead.

(B), (C), (D) The mean spatial initial .04 vector is rotated approximately 40° posteriorly because there is an initial negative deflection of .04 second duration in Leads V-1, V-2, V-3 and an initial positive deflection in Leads V-5 and V-6. (The initial .04 second appears re-sultantly zero in V-4.) The mean ST vector is rotated approximately 80° anteriorly since the ST segment is elevated in Leads V-1, V-2, V-3, V-4, V-5. The mean T vector is rotated 45° posteriorly because the transitional pathway for the T wave passes between electrode positions V-4 and V-5.

(E) Final summary figure illustrating the spatial arrangement of the vectors. The mean initial .04 vector is rotated to the left and abnormally posteriorly, pointing away from the anterodiaphragmatic region of the left ventricle. The QS deflections in Lead III and aV_F suggest the pattern of an inferior myocardial infarction and the absent initial R waves in V-1, V-2, V-3 suggest an anteroseptal infarction. One dead zone can produce such an electrocardiogram and one need not postulate two myocardial infarctions. The mean spatial ST vector is directed toward an area of anterodiaphragmatic epicardial injury.

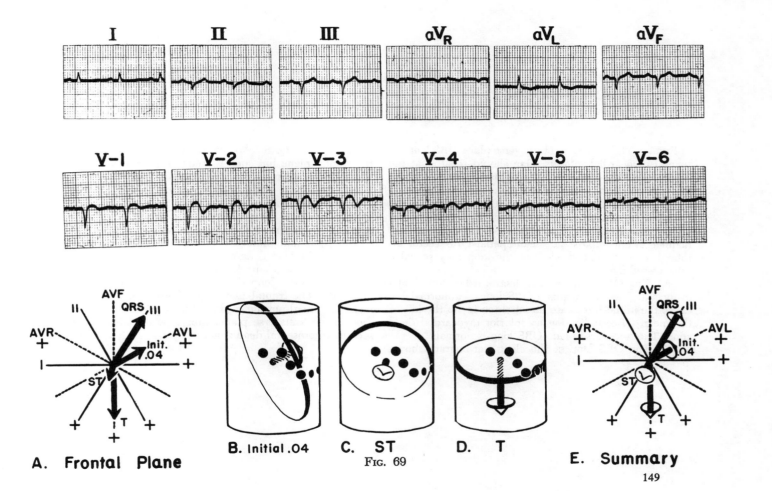

I II III aV_R aV_L aV_F

V-1 V-2 V-3 V-4 V-5 V-6

A. Frontal Plane   B. Initial .04   C. ST   D. T   E. Summary

FIG. 69

149

Fig. 70. The frontal and transverse plane QRS loops of several myocardial infarcts. One should recall that the QRS loop in the normal subject is narrow and elongate (fig. 24). Normally the initial forces are anterior to and relatively parallel with the mean QRS vector. In the normal subject a line drawn through the termini of the instantaneous vectors passes in a smooth and orderly manner to encompass the mean spatial QRS vector although one or another view of the loop may reveal a crisscrossed figure.

(A) The QRS loop of the electrocardiogram shown in fig. 58. The frontal plane QRS loop is abnormal because the initial forces are directed too far to the left of the mean QRS, indicating an inferior myocardial dead zone. The transverse plane QRS loop is normal.

(B) The QRS loop of the electrocardiogram shown in fig. 61. The QRS loop crosses itself when viewed in the frontal plane but such is frequently seen normally. The initial portion of the QRS loop is deformed as seen in the transverse plane and indicates an anteroseptal myocardial dead zone.

(C) The QRS loop of the electrocardiogram shown in fig. 66. The entire QRS loop is located abnormally to the right and markedly posteriorly and the initial portion of the loop is deformed. This type of loop indicates an extensive anterior myocardial dead zone.

(D) The QRS loop of the electrocardiogram shown in fig. 68. The frontal plane QRS loop is entirely normal. The initial portion of the QRS loop is deformed as seen in the transverse plane. This type of deformity is seen in anteroseptal dead zone.

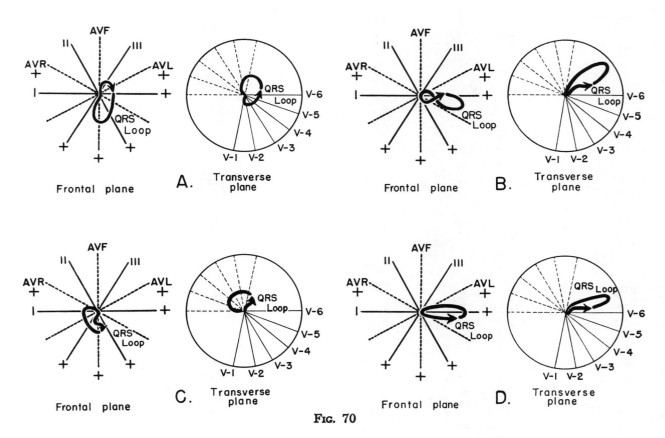

Frontal plane

A. Transverse plane

Frontal plane

B. Transverse plane

Frontal plane

C. Transverse plane

Frontal plane

D. Transverse plane

FIG. 70

CHAPTER FIVE

Intraventricular Conduction Abnormalities

Normal Ventricular Conduction and Depolarization

The propagating impulse from the A-V node and bundle of His is delivered to the ventricular muscle cells by way of the specialized intraventricular conducting system. This system is composed of the right and left bundle branches, their peripheral ramifications, and transitional cells which are anatomically and physiologically intermediate between the specialized conducting cells and ordinary muscle cells. The right bundle branch is a thin, long solitary structure running down the right septal surface from base toward apex, fanning out into peripheral ramifications distal to the base of the anteroseptal papillary muscle. The left bundle branch originates as a more broad sheet of fibers entering the left ventricle through the membranous portion of the septum under the aortic ring and branching early into two collections of fibers, the anterior (superior) and posterior (inferior) divisions of the left bundle branch. The anterior division courses toward the anterolateral papillary muscle and the posterior toward the posteromedial papillary muscle. Thus, from an anatomic and, as discussed below, from a pathophysiologic point of view, the intraventricular conducting system may be conceived as a *trifascicular* structure: (1) the right bundle branch; (2) the anterior division of the left bundle branch; and (3) the posterior division of the left bundle branch.

The earliest site of coupling between specialized conducting tissue and ordinary muscle in the normal adult subject appears to occur on the mid-left septal endocardium. Simultaneously, two other endocardial sites (probably in the distribution of the anterior and posterior

153

divisions) are depolarized, and the three areas rapidly merge on the endocardial surface. Within .01 to .02 second an endocardial site in the right ventricular apex begins to be depolarized, but the earlier left septal depolarization sets the stage for the vector of activity to progress from the left septum toward the right. Most of the septum is depolarized within the first .02 to .03 second, with the apex being depolarized before the base. Following the initial .04 second, which roughly represents septal and endocardial depolarization, the remaining forces generated during the QRS cycle are produced by depolarization of the deeper and epicardial regions of the ventricular musculature. The left ventricle is normally thicker than the right and the electrical forces generated by the left ventricle dominate the electrical field during the major portion of the remaining QRS cycle. As depolarization spreads through the ventricular walls it reaches the epicardium of a low anterior region of the right ventricle first. Following this, the wave of depolarization reaches the apical epicardium of the left ventricle. As succeeding epicardial regions of the left ventricle are depolarized, the

mean electrical vector at the given instant of depolarization points more and more leftward and posteriorly. The basal portion of the left ventricle is usually the last part of the ventricular musculature to undergo depolarization and the terminal forces are directed to the left and posteriorly.

In the normal subject the QRS interval, representing the duration of ventricular depolarization, is seldom more than .09 to .10 second, and often .08 second or less. When the QRS interval is .12 second or more, some form of bundle branch block is usually present. Ventricular hypertrophy may prolong the QRS duration but it is unlikely that hypertrophy alone prolongs the QRS beyond .12 second. In addition, abnormalities of conduction in one of the two divisions of the left bundle branch, and normal conduction in the other division as well as the right bundle branch, may produce abnormal conduction patterns, referred to as *hemiblocks* (see below), which are frequently characterized by QRS durations of .09 to .11 second in the presence of other evidence of abnormal sequences of depolarization. The sequence of ventricular depolarization in the normal adult subject is illustrated in fig. 71.

Right Bundle Branch Block

The Sequence of Depolarization When There Is Right Bundle Branch Block. When the right bundle branch is blocked or fails as a conduction pathway, the sequence of ventricular depolarization is altered. The left side of the ventricular septum undergoes depolarization first, just as when conduction was normal, but because the right bundle branch is blocked and left ventricular conduction pathways are normal, this brief septal event is immediately followed by depolarization of left ventricular musculature exclusively. Therefore, during the next few hundredths of a second the electrical field is dominated by left ventricular forces which are directed to the left and slightly posteriorly. Because the right bundle branch is blocked, right ventricular depolarization is delayed and does not begin to influence the electrical field for at least .04 second, the time it takes depolarization to spread across the septum. As the right ventricle is beginning to generate forces, the left ventricular forces are beginning to subside, and the instantaneous

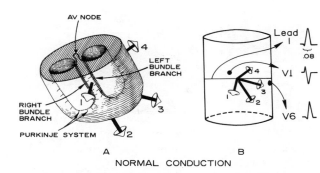

Fig. 71. The sequence of ventricular depolarization in the normal adult subject.

(A) The A-V node and right and left bundle branches are shown. Vector one is directed slightly to the right and anteriorly and is produced by depolarization of the septum from left to right, and adjacent regions of the endocardium. Forces produced by depolarization of the remaining endocardial regions, right ventricular, and apical left ventricular epicardial regions result in vector two. Vector three is the resultant of a large number of left ventricular myocardial forces and dwindling right ventricular forces. The resultant of such forces will be directed to the left and posteriorly. Vector four, produced almost entirely from the left ventricle, is directed to the left and posteriorly.

(B) This illustrates how the spatial vectors illustrated in (A) will influence Leads I, V-1, and V-6. These particular deflections are shown because the QRS contour exhibited by these leads is frequently used to determine whether right or left bundle branch block is present and to estimate the direction of septal depolarization.

155

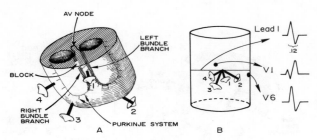

RIGHT BUNDLE BRANCH SYSTEM

Fig. 72. The sequence of depolarization when there is right bundle branch block.

(A) Vector one, resulting from septal and left ventricular endocardial depolarization, is directed slightly to the left and anteriorly. Vector two is produced by depolarization of the left ventricular musculature and is directed to the left and slightly posteriorly. Vector three is the resultant of a large number of right ventricular forces and a smaller number of left ventricular forces. The resultant of such forces is directed to the right and anteriorly. Vector four, produced almost entirely by the right ventricle, is directed more to the right and anteriorly.

(B) This illustrates how the spatial vectors illustrated in (A) will influence Leads I, V-1, and V-6. Note how the spatial vectors in right bundle branch block produce a quite specific deflection contour pattern characterized by a broad S wave in Leads I and V-6 and a small initial R wave followed by an S wave and larger terminal R wave in Lead V-1. The QRS duration is .12 second. Vector four is directed toward the right and anteriorly, demonstrating that the terminal forces are generated from the right ventricle.

156

QRS vectors begin to drift slowly to the right and anteriorly. Accordingly, since the last portion of the cardiac muscle to undergo depolarization in this circumstance is the right ventricle, the terminal instantaneous QRS vectors are directed to the right and anteriorly in right bundle branch block. The sequence of depolarization when there is right bundle branch block is illustrated in fig. 72.

The Mean Spatial Terminal .04 Vector. This vector represents the mean of all forces generated during the terminal .04 portion of the QRS cycle, and is directed toward the blocked ventricle when bundle branch block is present. Accordingly, when there is right bundle branch block, the terminal .04 vector is directed to the right and is usually anteriorly directed as well.

Duration of the QRS Complexes. When right bundle branch block is present, the QRS duration is usually prolonged to .12 second or longer. The widest QRS complex should be used to determine the QRS duration.

Direction of the Mean Spatial T Vector. When the sequence of ventricular depolarization is altered, the sequence of repolarization is changed. Therefore in bundle branch block, the mean spatial T vector is directed opposite to the mean spatial QRS vector and the QRS-T angle approaches 180°.

When the bundle branch block is uncomplicated; that is, when bundle block is the only lesion, the ventricular gradient is normal; but when local ventricular ischemia is also present, the ventricular gradient may become abnormal.

Direction of the Mean Spatial ST Vector. A prominent ST vector is usually present in right bundle branch block and represents early forces of repolarization. This vector is usually relatively parallel with the mean T vector. When the mean ST vector is large and is not relatively parallel with the mean T vector, another lesion, perhaps the myocardial injury of coronary occlusion, should be considered.

Right Bundle Branch Block Combined with Other Lesions. The dead zone effect of myocardial infarction will alter the QRS loop of right bundle branch block in the same way that it alters the loop when conduction is normal. This can occur because left ventricular depolarization occurs in a normal manner in uncomplicated right bundle branch block, and most infarcts occur in the left ventricle, thereby altering left ventricular depolarization.

Etiology of Right Bundle Branch Block. The most frequent cause of right bundle branch block is coronary arteriosclerosis. This type of block also may be associated with interventricular and interatrial septal defect, and may occur transiently during pulmonary embolism. It may result from various forms of conducting system fibrosis, myocarditis, and cardiomyopathies. It may also occur in combination with block in the anterior division of the left bundle branch, thereby producing abnormal left axis deviation in combination with the right bundle branch block as a result of conducting system fibrosis and coronary atherosclerosis. This pattern may also appear in certain congenital defects such as atrial septal defects of the primum type and endocardial cushion defects. The combination of right bundle branch block and block of the posterior division of the left bundle may be indicated by a right bundle pattern combined with abnormal right axis deviation. Physiological right bundle branch block is occasionally asso-

157

ciated with increased heart rate. The rate need not be excessive in some subjects. Apparently this type of block is the result of bundle "fatigue" in a susceptible subject. Similarly, functional right bundle branch block commonly occurs during conduction of early premature supraventricular beats, especially when the preceding cycle is long (see Chapter 15). Right bundle branch block may occur in young subjects with no history or evidence of heart disease and may represent a congenital defect of the conduction system. The etiology of right bundle branch block must be determined clinically.

The following electrocardiograms (figs. 73 and 74) are examples of right bundle branch block.

FIG. 73. The electrocardiogram of a hypertensive patient, 63 years of age, showing right bundle branch block.

(A) Frontal plane projection of the mean QRS, T, and terminal .04 vectors. In this case there is a deep S wave in Lead I and the terminal .04 second of the QRS complex in Lead aV_F is resultantly zero. Therefore the terminal .04 vector is directed to the right and is perpendicular to Lead aV_F.

(B) The terminal .04 vector is approximately flush with the frontal plane because the transitional pathway for the terminal .04 vector passes between V-1 and V-2. The terminal .04 portion of the QRS complex is positive in Lead V-1 but negative in V-2, V-3, V-4, V-5, and V-6.

(C) The mean QRS vector is approximately flush with the frontal plane since the QRS complex is resultantly positive in V-1 but resultantly negative in the remaining precordial leads.

(D) The mean T vector is flush with the frontal plane since the transitional pathway for the T wave passes through electrode position V-2.

(E) Final summary figure showing the spatial arrangement of the vectors. The QRS duration is .12 second, indicating bundle branch block. The terminal .04 vector is directed to the right and indicates right bundle branch block.

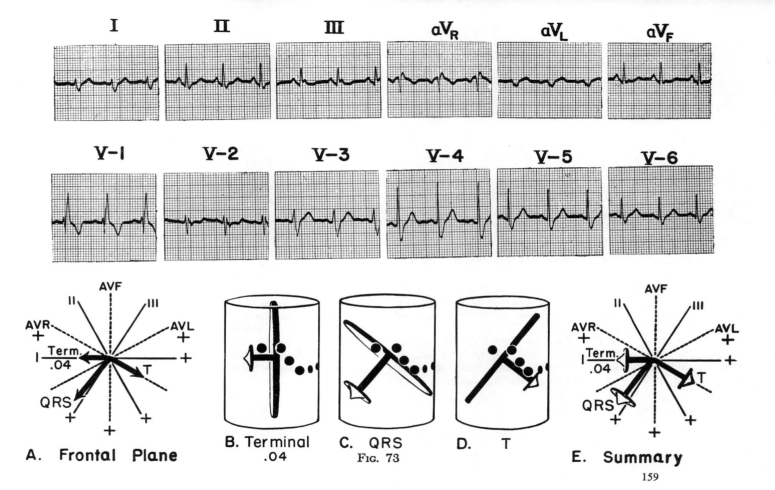

I II III aV$_R$ aV$_L$ aV$_F$

V-1 V-2 V-3 V-4 V-5 V-6

A. Frontal Plane

B. Terminal .04

C. QRS

FIG. 73

D. T

E. Summary

159

Fig. 74. The electrocardiogram of a patient, 60 years of age, showing posterior myocardial infarction and right bundle branch block.

(A) The frontal plane projection of the mean QRS, ST, T, and terminal .04 vectors. Note that the last .04 second of the QRS complex is large and negative in Leads I and II and slightly positive in Lead III and slightly negative in Lead aV_L. This portion of the QRS complexes can be represented by a vector located between the negative limb of Lead I and the positive limb of Lead aV_R.

(B) The terminal .04 vector is rotated approximately 20° anteriorly because the last portion of the QRS complex is positive in V-1 and V-2 and negative in Leads V-3, V-4, V-5, V-6.

(C) The mean QRS vector is rotated approximately 30° anteriorly, producing resultantly positive QRS deflections in all the precordial leads. Note how Leads V-4, V-5, V-6 are recording near the transitional pathway and that these complexes are resultantly less positive than the complexes recorded from the remaining precordial leads.

(D) The mean ST vector is rotated slightly posteriorly and the mean T vector is rotated slightly anteriorly.

(E) Summary. The QRS duration is .13 second, indicating bundle branch block. The terminal .04 QRS vector is directed to the right and anteriorly, indicating right bundle branch block. The QRS-T angle is in an abnormal position because the mean QRS and T vectors are located above the Lead I axis. (To be discussed later.) The T vector is directed away from an area of diaphragmatic ischemia. There is a prominent ST vector present directed toward the inferior surface of the heart identifying epicardial injury in that region. This electrocardiogram illustrates the simultaneous occurrence of right bundle branch block and posterior myocardial infarction.

160

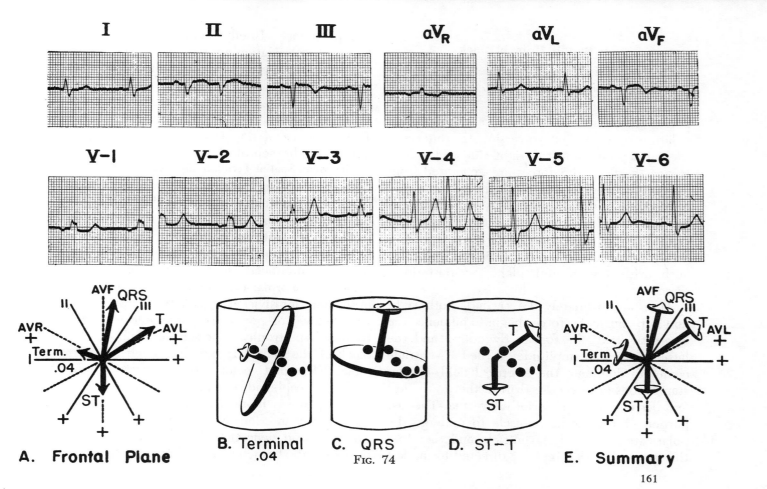

I II III aV$_R$ aV$_L$ aV$_F$

V-1 V-2 V-3 V-4 V-5 V-6

A. Frontal Plane

B. Terminal .04

C. QRS

D. ST-T

E. Summary

Fig. 74

161

Left Bundle Branch Block

The Sequence of Depolarization When There Is Left Bundle Branch Block. When complete block of the main left bundle branch is present, depolarization can reach the left ventricular musculature only by first traversing the interventricular septum from the right side to the left. Hence the first QRS forces are generated from the right ventricle and from the septum. Accordingly, their direction will vary with the thickness and lie of the septum and thickness of the right ventricle. The initial QRS forces are usually directed to the left and anteriorly but may be flush with the frontal plane or posteriorly directed.

After approximately .04 second, both right and left ventricular forces begin to influence the electrical field, the former dwindling and the latter growing in amplitude. As the left ventricle comes to dominate the electrical field, the instantaneous QRS vectors drift farther to the left and become more posteriorly directed. The last portion of the cardiac muscle to undergo depolarization is the left ventricle and therefore the terminal QRS forces are directed to the left

and posteriorly. Briefly then, the left ventricle begins depolarization approximately .04 second after the right ventricle and right ventricular depolarization is completed before that of the left ventricle, leaving purely left ventricular terminal forces to dominate the electrical field. The sequence of depolarization when there is left bundle branch block is illustrated in fig. 75.

The Mean Spatial Terminal .04 Vector. This vector represents the mean of all forces generated during the terminal .04 second of the QRS cycle. The terminal .04 second vector is usually directed to the left and posteriorly when there is left bundle branch block because the terminal forces are produced exclusively by the left ventricle. If abnormal conduction in the radiation of the anterior division of the left bundle branch (see below) or perhaps considerable left ventricular hypertrophy is present, combined with block of the main left bundle branch, the terminal .04 second vector may be directed cephalad. This cephalad or superior deviation in the frontal plane is more marked in the setting of block of the anterior division. In some cases, the standard lead deflections look like the pattern of left bundle branch block or left anterior hemiblock (see below), and the precordial lead deflections look like the pattern of right bundle branch block. In a variant of this pattern, complete left bundle branch block and right bundle branch block alternate in time. Both of these are generally associated with fibrosis in the region of the proximal intraventricular conducting system and probably represent so-called bilateral bundle branch block. It appears to be a forerunner of complete heart block (see Chapter 17).

Duration of the QRS Complexes. When left bundle branch block is present, the QRS duration is prolonged to .12 second or longer. The widest QRS complex should be used to determine the QRS duration.

Direction of the Mean Spatial T Vector. When the sequence of ventricular depolarization is altered, the sequence of repolarization is changed. Thus, in left bundle branch block, the mean T vector is directed opposite to the mean QRS vector and the QRS-T angle approaches 180°. When left bundle branch block is uncomplicated, that is, when left bundle block is the only lesion, the ventricular gradient is normal. But when a significant amount of ventricular

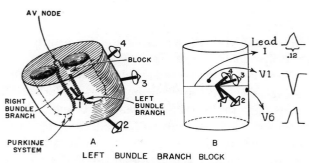

Fig. 75. The sequence of depolarization when there is left bundle branch block.

(A) Vector one, resulting from septal and right ventricular endocardial depolarization, is directed slightly to the left and is flush with the frontal plane. Vector two is produced by right and left ventricular depolarization and is directed to the left and posteriorly. Vector three is produced by a large number of left ventricular forces and a smaller number of right ventricular forces. The resultant of such forces is directed to the left and posteriorly. Vector four, produced almost entirely by the left ventricle, is directed to the left and posteriorly.

(B) This illustrates how the spatial vectors illustrated in (A) will influence Leads I, V-1, and V-6. Note how the spatial vectors explain the typical "pattern" of left bundle branch block characterized by a broad slurred R wave in Lead I and V-6 and a broad negative deflection in V-1. The QRS duration is at least .12 second. The last vector of the QRS loop is directed toward the left and posteriorly pointing toward the left ventricle and therefore indicates that the left bundle branch is blocked.

163

ischemia is also present, the ventricular gradient may become abnormal.

Direction of the Mean Spatial ST Vector. A prominent ST vector representing early repolarization is usually present in left bundle branch block. The vector representing ST-segment displacement usually lies relatively parallel with the mean T vector. When the mean ST vector is large and is not relatively parallel with the mean T vector, another lesion, perhaps myocardial injury or coronary occlusion, should be considered.

Left Bundle Branch Block and Myocardial Infarction. Left bundle branch block usually obscures the QRS abnormality of myocardial infarction. This is understandable when one recalls that the initial forces in left bundle branch block result from the depolarization of the ventricular septum and the right ventricle. These early forces would not be disturbed in myocardial infarction, then, unless the dead zone includes a large portion of the interventricular septum. Ordinarily in left bundle branch block the initial QRS forces are directed to the left, and one rarely sees a Q wave in Lead I. When a large

septal infarction has occurred, the initial QRS forces may be directed abnormally to the right, producing a Q wave in Lead I, which is often diagnostic of myocardial infarction in left bundle branch block. Likewise, when the anterior portion of the ventricular septum has been destroyed by infarction, the initial QRS forces may be directed markedly posteriorly and abnormal Q waves may be recorded in the precordial leads. When there is uncomplicated left bundle branch block, the mean ST vector is relatively parallel with the mean T vector. However, when the mean ST vector is 100° or more away from the mean T vector, one should suspect epicardial injury due to myocardial infarction. Another way to identify myocardial infarction in the presence of left bundle branch block, as has been mentioned, is to see if the ventricular gradient is abnormally directed by the epicardial ischemia associated with coronary occlusion. Of course, a normal ventricular gradient by no means rules out a myocardial infarction.

Etiology of Left Bundle Branch Block. The most common causes of left bundle branch block are coronary atherosclerosis with or without the *clinical* symptoms of coronary disease, or fibrosis of the proximal conducting system. This type of bundle block only rarely occurs as a result of congenital heart disease, but may be associated with many types of cardiomyopathies or of myocarditis. Functional left bundle branch block, dependent upon rate, may also occur. The exact etiology and significance of left bundle branch block must be determined clinically.

The following electrocardiograms (figs. 76 and 77) are examples of left bundle branch block.

Block in the Divisions of the Left Bundle Branch: The Hemiblocks

As described earlier, the main left bundle branch is a short structure which divides on the left interventricular septum into two major collections of fibers, forming an anterior (or superior) division and a posterior (or inferior) division. Disease in the radiations of either of these two divisions may produce abnormal patterns of depolarization of the left ventricular musculature.

The Pure Hemiblocks. The abnormal patterns in hemiblocks result from delayed excitation of those portions of the myocardium served by the affected division. Since only one of the two left bundle branch divisions is involved in this setting, the resulting electrocardiographic pattern is called a "hemiblock." The hemiblocks differ from typical left bundle branch block (see above) in two major ways: (1) the QRS duration in pure hemiblock is usually .10 second or less, whereas it is usually .12 second or more in complete bundle branch block; and (2) the mean QRS axis is usually —60° or more in left anterior hemiblock and at least +120° or more in left posterior hemiblock, whereas it is usually normal in pure complete left bundle branch block. Therefore, in pure left anterior hemiblock, the mean initial .04 second vector is inferior (or horizontal) and to the left, and the terminal .04 second vector is superior and to the left (fig. 78). Conversely, in pure left posterior hemiblock the mean initial .04 second vector is oriented superiorly or slightly inferiorly and to the left or slightly to the right, while the mean terminal .04 second vector is oriented more to the right and inferiorly.

Combined Block in the Right Branch or Main Left Bundle Branch and the Anterior or Posterior Division of the Left Bundle Branch. It is generally accepted that pure right bundle branch block

Fig. 76. The electrocardiogram of a clinically normal 44-year-old male, showing left bundle branch block.

(A) The frontal plane projection of the mean QRS, T, and terminal .04 vectors. Note that the terminal portion of the QRS complex is positive in Lead II and negative in Lead III and aV$_F$. This terminal .04 second of the QRS complex can be represented by a mean vector located between the positive limb of Lead I and aV$_L$.

(B) The terminal .04 QRS vector is tilted approximately 40° posteriorly because that portion of the QRS complex is negative in Leads V-1, V-2, V-3 and positive in Leads V-5, V-6.

(C) The mean QRS vector is rotated approximately 30° posteriorly because the transitional pathway passes between electrode positions V-3 and V-4.

(D) The mean T vector is rotated approximately 30° anteriorly because all the precordial T waves are positive and the T wave in V-1 is only slightly larger than the T wave in V-6.

(E) Summary. The QRS duration is .13 second, indicating bundle branch block. The terminal .04 vector is directed to the left and posteriorly pointing toward the left ventricle and therefore indicates left bundle branch block.

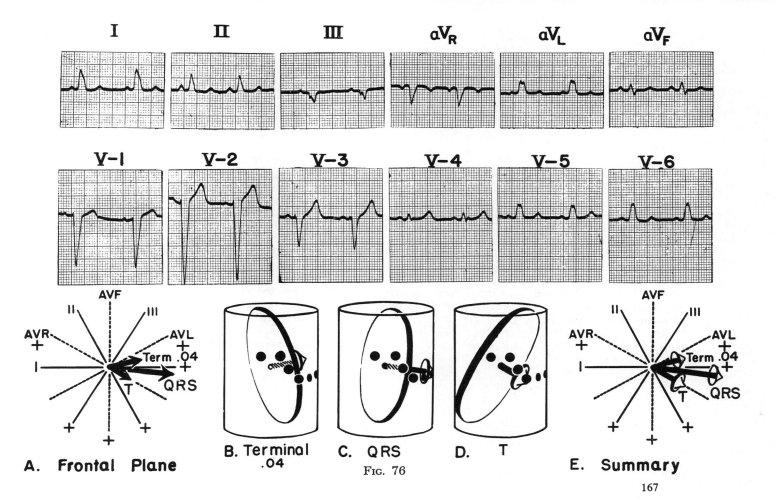

I II III aV_R aV_L aV_F

V-1 V-2 V-3 V-4 V-5 V-6

A. Frontal Plane

B. Terminal .04

C. QRS

D. T

E. Summary

Fig. 76

Fig. 77. The electrocardiogram of a hypertensive patient showing left bundle branch block and extensive anterior myocardial ischemia.

(A) The frontal plane projection of the mean QRS, T, and terminal .04 vectors.

(B) The terminal .04 vector is directed approximately 60° posteriorly since the terminal portion of the QRS complex is negative in V-1, V-2, V-3, V-4, and is positive in V-5 and V-6.

(C) The mean QRS vector is rotated approximately 50° posteriorly because the transitional pathway passes between electrode positions V-4 and V-5.

(D) The mean T vector is rotated approximately 50° posteriorly since the T waves are inverted in V-1, V-2, V-3, V-4, and upright in V-5 and V-6.

(E) Summary. The QRS duration is .16 second in V-3 and is approximately .12 second in all of the extremity leads, suggesting that a certain portion of the terminal QRS forces is relatively perpendicular to the frontal plane. The terminal .04 vector is directed to the left and posteriorly, indicating left bundle branch block. The mean T vector is directed abnormally posteriorly away from the anterior surface of the heart and indicates anterior myocardial ischemia. The mean T vector is almost always directed anteriorly in uncomplicated bundle branch block and can be considered abnormal when directed posteriorly. In this case the enclosed QRS-T angle lies posteriorly and therefore the ventricular gradient is directed abnormally posteriorly.

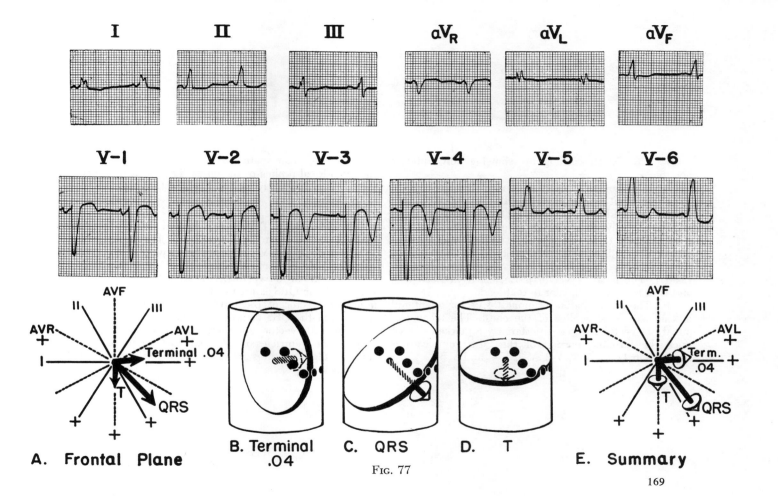

I II III aV_R aV_L aV_F

V-1 V-2 V-3 V-4 V-5 V-6

A. Frontal Plane

B. Terminal .04

C. QRS

D. T

E. Summary

Fig. 77

169

Fig. 78. Electrocardiogram showing left anterior hemiblock.

(A) The frontal plane projection of the mean QRS, T, and terminal .04 vectors. The QRS complex is slightly positive in Lead aV_R and is largest and negative in Lead III. Accordingly, the mean QRS vector is drawn almost perpendicular to lead axis aV_R. The terminal .04 portion of the QRS complex represented as a mean vector is isoelectric in Lead I and is drawn perpendicular to Lead I. The mean T vector is isoelectric in Lead aV_L and is drawn perpendicular to that lead.

(B) The mean spatial terminal .04 vector orientated in the cylindrical replica of the chest. The mean terminal .04 vector is rotated posteriorly a marked degree since the terminal portion of the QRS complexes is negative in Leads V-1, V-2, V-3, V-4, and V-5.

(C) The mean spatial QRS vector is orientated in the cylindrical replica of the chest. The mean QRS vector is rotated slightly posterior since the edge of the transitional pathway which is perpendicular to the vector lies close to V-4.

(D) The mean T vector is rotated anteriorly to a marked degree since the T waves are positive in Leads V-1, V-2, V-3, and V-4, but are negative in Lead V-6.

(E) Final summary illustrating the mean spatial QRS, T, and terminal .04 vectors. Note that the left axis deviation of the QRS is greater than $-60°$; that the terminal .04 vector of the QRS is $-90°$; and that the duration of the QRS complexes is normal (.08 second). The initial .04 vector representing the initial depolarization of the ventricles is directed to the left and inferiorly. These features are characteristic of left anterior hemiblock.

170

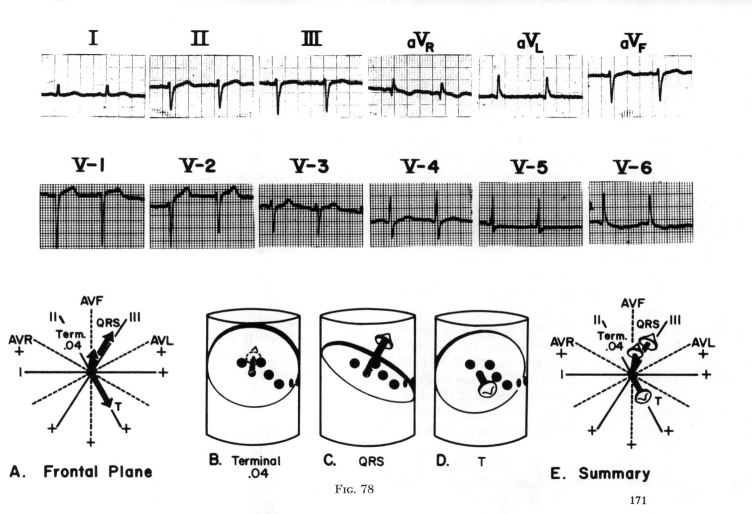

I II III aV_R aV_L aV_F

V-1 V-2 V-3 V-4 V-5 V-6

A. Frontal Plane

B. Terminal .04

C. QRS

D. T

E. Summary

Fig. 78

171

produces no significant leftward change in the mean QRS vector. When right bundle branch block is combined with abnormal left axis deviation, therefore, it is assumed that the right bundle branch block is combined with left anterior hemiblock (fig. 79). When pre-existing right bundle branch is accompanied by a rightward shift of the mean frontal QRS axis, in the absence of clinical right ventricular hypertrophy, coexistant left posterior hemiblock may be present (fig. 80). In either instance, the combination of right bundle branch block and block of one of the divisions of the left bundle branch is referred to as *bifascicular block*.

Since left anterior hemiblock causes abnormal left axis deviation, and complete left bundle branch block usually does not produce abnormal mean frontal QRS axis shifts, the combination of complete left bundle branch block and abnormal left axis deviation may indicate block at the level of the main left bundle branch combined with abnormal conduction in the radiation of the anterior division of the left bundle branch (see fig. 81).

Trifascicular Block. The combination of high grade or complete block in the right bundle branch and one of the divisions of the left bundle branch, along with delay in the other division of the left bundle branch, is referred to as *trifascicular block*. It is suggested electrocardiographically by tracings such as figs. 79 and 80 in combination with a prolonged P-R interval. The latter suggests slowed (abnormal) conduction in the third fascicle, but can only be proved by intracardiac catheter recordings of His bundle activity.

Etiology and Complications of the Hemiblocks

The etiology of the hemiblocks is still uncertain. They may occur secondary to conduction system disease, such as described by Lev and Lenegre, as well as coronary atherosclerosis. Trifascicular block frequently progresses to complete heart disease and bifascicular block may also progress.

S_1, S_2, S_3 Pattern

In most normal subjects the basal portion of the left ventricle is last to undergo depolarization. Therefore the terminal QRS forces are directed to the left and posteriorly. In an occasional normal subject the right ventricle contributes large terminal forces which are directed to the right and may be anterior or posterior to or flush with the frontal plane. Unlike bundle branch block the QRS duration is not prolonged. In such cases the QRS loop is not elongated as it usually is but is wide and bean-shaped. Since the QRS loop is bean-shaped, it produces positive and negative deflections on many of the limb and precordial leads, frequently resulting in S waves in Leads I, II, III, and many of the precordial leads. In some cases the R and S waves are of the same amplitude in nearly all leads. Under such circumstances it is often very difficult and of little value to plot a mean QRS vector. The exact cause of this unusual sequence of depolarization is not known, and perhaps there are multiple causes. Some have felt that the thick muscular ridge known as the crista supraventricularis is the source of rightward terminal QRS forces, and others have suggested that a QRS loop of this sort results from a congenital defect of the Purkinje system.

The S_1, S_2, S_3 pattern is one electrocardiographic syndrome where a wide spatial QRS-T angle is encountered with a QRS interval that is normal. The ventricular gradient is normal because the mean T vector is frequently increased in magnitude and normal in direction.

The electrocardiogram shown in fig. 82 is an example of the S_1, S_2, S_3 pattern.

The Pre-Excitation Syndromes

Under normal conditions, as well as in most abnormal states, the cardiac impulse propagating from the atria is delivered to the ventricles by way of the A-V node, the His bundle, and the intraventricular conducting system. The time required for the impulse to traverse this pathway accounts for the normal atrioventricular conduction time, or electrocardiographically, the P-R interval (see Chapters 11 and 17). When tracts of ordinary muscle or specialized conducting tissue are available to bypass all of, or parts of, this normal pathway, early excitation of parts of the ventricular myocardium may occur. If the bypass tracts enter ventricular muscle remote from the specialized conducting system, an initial vector demonstrating slow muscle conduction and a short P-R interval will be present. This form of pre-excitation is known as the Wolff-Parkinson-White syndrome, and the

Fig. 79. The electrocardiogram of a hypertensive patient, 76 years of age, showing right bundle branch block and left anterior hemiblock.

(A) The frontal plane projection of the mean QRS, T, and terminal .04 vectors. The terminal .04 portion of the QRS complex is markedly negative in Lead I and isoelectric in Lead aV_F. The mean vector representing this portion of the QRS complex would be directed perpendicular to Lead aV_F and toward the negative pole of Lead I.

(B) The terminal .04 vector is rotated 30° anteriorly because this portion of the QRS complexes is positive in V-1 and V-2 and negative in V-4, V-5, V-6.

(C) The mean QRS vector is rotated 30° anteriorly because the transitional pathway passes between electrode positions V-3 and V-4. In such a case V-1, V-2, V-3 will record resultantly positive deflections and V-4, V-5, V-6 will record resultantly negative deflections.

(D) The mean T vector is rotated 15° posteriorly because the transitional pathway for the T wave is located between electrode positions V-2 and V-3.

(E) Summary. The QRS duration is .12 second. The terminal .04 vector is directed to the right and anteriorly, indicating right bundle branch block. The mid-portion of the QRS is directed markedly superiorly, suggesting block in the anterior division of the left bundle branch.

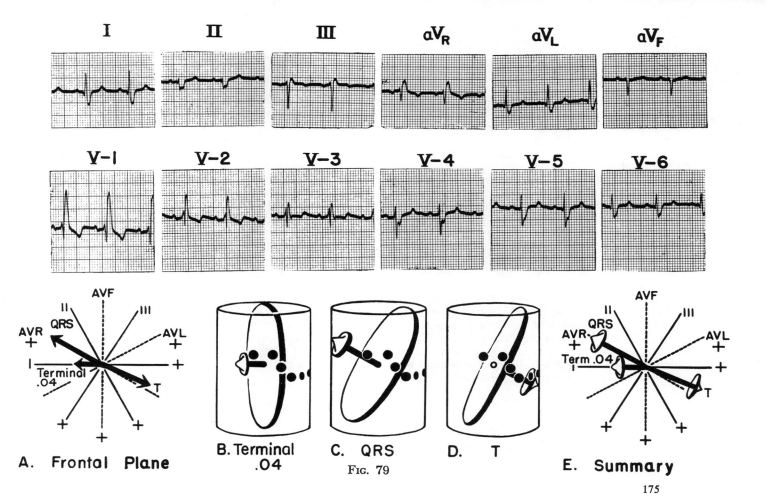

I II III aV_R aV_L aV_F

V-1 V-2 V-3 V-4 V-5 V-6

A. Frontal Plane

B. Terminal .04

C. QRS

D. T

Fig. 79

E. Summary

175

FIG. 80. Electrocardiogram showing right bundle branch block and probable left posterior hemiblock. An earlier electrocardiogram showed right bundle branch block with a normal QRS axis.

(A) The frontal plane projection of the mean spatial QRS, T, and terminal .04 QRS vectors. The QRS complex is slightly positive in Lead aV_F and is negative in Lead I. Therefore the QRS is almost perpendicular to lead axis aV_F. The T wave is slightly positive in Lead III and aV_L. Therefore the mean T vector is located as shown. The mean vector representing the terminal .04 portion of the QRS is directed to the right and is nearly perpendicular to lead axis aV_F because the terminal .04 portion of the QRS is small but negative in aV_F and positive in Lead III.

(B) The mean spatial terminal .04 vector orientated in the cylindrical replica of the chest. The mean terminal .04 vector is flush with the frontal plane because the terminal .04 portion of the QRS is positive in Lead V-1 and negative in V-2, and the edge of transitional pathway, which is perpendicular to the vector, must pass between these two electrode positions.

(C) The mean QRS vector orientated in the cylindrical replica of the chest. The mean QRS vector is flush with the frontal plane because the edge of the transitional pathway must pass between electrode position V-1 where the QRS complex is positive and V-2 where it is slightly negative.

(D) The mean T vector orientated in the cylindrical replica of the chest. The edge of the transitional pathway of the mean T vector must pass between electrode positions V-3 and V-4 since the T wave is negative in V-3 and positive in V-4. Since the transitional pathway is perpendicular to the vector, it follows that the mean T vector must be rotated slightly posteriorly to meet the conditions described.

(E) Final summary figure illustrating the mean spatial QRS, T, and terminal .04 vectors. Note that the QRS is .12 second in duration and that the mean QRS and terminal .04 second vectors are directed far to the right. These characteristics suggest right bundle branch block plus left posterior hemiblock, since earlier tracings had shown right bundle branch block with a normal axis.

176

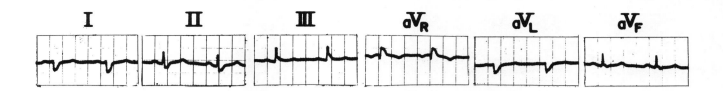

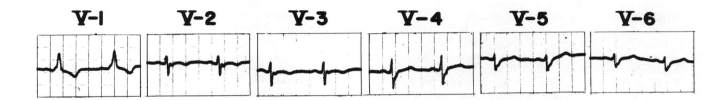

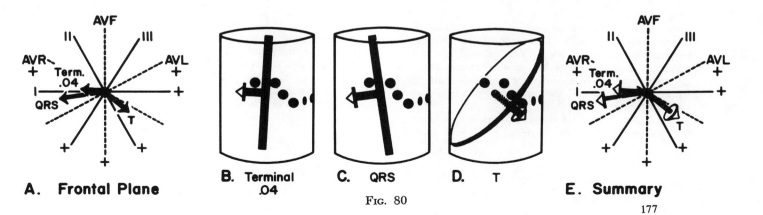

A. Frontal Plane

B. Terminal .04

C. QRS

D. T

E. Summary

Fig. 80

177

Fig. 81. The electrocardiogram of a 50-year-old male who had a classical clinical picture of myocardial infarction illustrating how left bundle branch block can mask the findings of myocardial infarction.

(A) Frontal plane projection of the mean spatial QRS, ST, T, and terminal .04 vectors. Note that the direction of the initial .04 vector is normal, that is, the initial deflection of the QRS complex is positive in Lead I and II and V-1 through V-6. The terminal .04 portion of the QRS complex is negative in Leads II, III, and aV$_F$ and approaches resultant zero in aV$_R$. (Note that the P-R interval in Lead II is .16 second and the QRS duration is .16 second. The P-R interval in Lead aV$_R$ is also .16 second but the QRS interval is only .12 second. This suggests that the terminal portion of Lead aV$_R$ is almost isoelectric and can be represented by a vector perpendicular to Lead aV$_R$.) This marked left axis deviation in the presence of left bundle branch block suggests the possibility of coexistent conduction abnormality in the radiation of the anterior division of the left bundle branch.

(B) The terminal .04 vector is rotated approximately 60° posteriorly since the terminal portion of the QRS complex is negative in Leads V-1, V-2, V-3, V-4, V-5, and is positive in V-6.

(C) The mean QRS vector is rotated approximately 50° posteriorly because the transitional pathway passes between electrode positions V-4 and V-5.

(D) The mean T vector is rotated approximately 75° anteriorly.

(E) Summary. The QRS duration of .16 second indicates bundle branch block. The terminal .04 vector is directed to the left and posteriorly indicating left bundle branch block. A prominent ST vector is present but because it is relatively parallel with the mean T vector it probably represents early repolarization. The ST segment displacement can become quite marked in bundle branch block and does not necessarily indicate myocardial infarction. The patient had a myocardial infarction several months before the electrocardiogram shown above was made. Left bundle branch block may completely obscure the QRS, ST, and T abnormalities. The abnormal left axis deviation suggests the possibility of abnormal conduction in the anterior division (i.e., hemiblock) combined with main left bundle branch block.

178

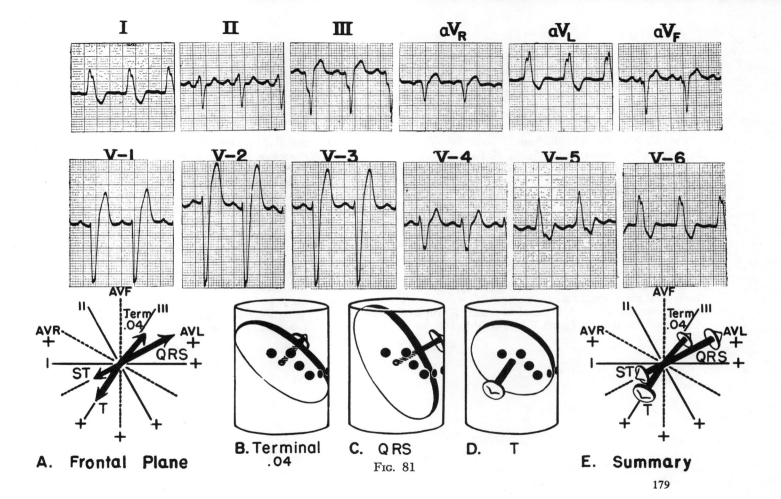

I   II   III   aV_R   aV_L   aV_F

V-1   V-2   V-3   V-4   V-5   V-6

A. Frontal Plane

B. Terminal .04

C. QRS

D. T

E. Summary

FIG. 81

Fig. 82. The electrocardiogram of a normal subject, 24 years of age, showing the S_1, S_2, S_3 pattern.

(A) Frontal plane projection of the initial and terminal .04 vectors and the mean T vector. Note that all the QRS complexes are approximately equiphasic in the standard and unipolar extremity leads. The initial .04 vector is slightly positive in Lead aV_L and the terminal .04 vector is resultantly zero in Lead aV_L. The initial .04 vector is directed toward the positive pole of Lead II and the terminal .04 vector is directed toward the negative pole of the same lead.

(B) The initial .04 vector is approximately flush with the frontal plane since there is an initial Q wave of .04 second duration in Lead V-1 and an initial R wave of .04 second duration in Leads V-3, V-4, V-5, V-6.

(C) The terminal .04 vector is directed approximately 15° posteriorly because terminal S waves are recorded in all of the precordial leads. Note that the transitional pathway for the terminal .04 vector lies very near electrode position V-1. Sometimes the terminal .04 vector is even more anteriorly directed with an R' at V-1 and even V-2.

(D) The mean T vector is rotated approximately 5° anteriorly since the transitional pathway is located between V-1 and V-2.

(E) Final summary figure. The QRS duration is only .08 to .09 second. The terminal portion of the QRS is located to the right and is directed slightly posteriorly. This type of tracing illustrates right ventricular conduction delay with normal QRS duration.

180

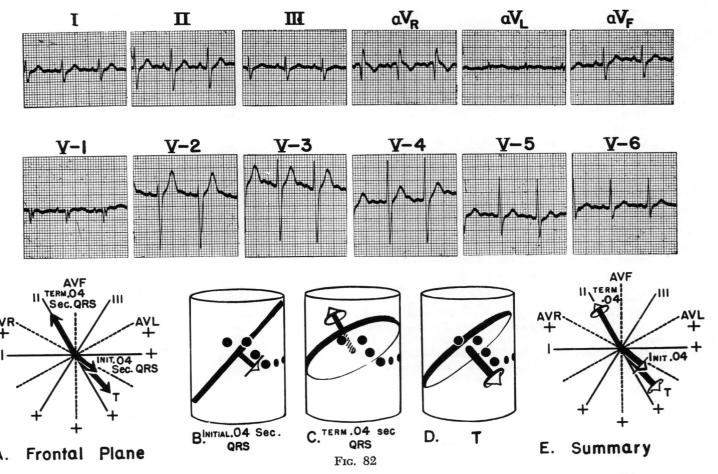

I   II   III   aV$_R$ aV$_L$ aV$_F$

V-1   V-2   V-3   V-4   V-5   V-6

A. Frontal Plane

B. INITIAL .04 Sec. QRS

C. TERM. .04 sec QRS

D. T

E. Summary

FIG. 82

181

Fig. 83A. Electrocardiogram showing type A Wolff-Parkinson-White conduction abnormality (pre-excitation syndrome).

(A) The frontal plane projection of the mean spatial QRS, ST, T, and delta wave vectors. The QRS complex is slightly negative to lead axis aV_F and is largest and positive in Lead I. This enables one to draw the mean QRS vector almost perpendicular to Lead aV_F. The T wave is largest in Lead II and slightly negative in Lead aV_L. This makes it possible to diagram the mean T vector almost parallel to Lead II. The delta wave—represented by the initial .04 portion of the QRS complex—is largest and negative in Lead III and is slightly negative in Lead II yet is resultantly negative in lead aV_R. This permits one to diagram the mean delta wave vector as illustrated.

(B) The mean spatial delta wave vector orientated in the cylindrical replica of the chest. The mean delta wave vector must be rotated anteriorly since the initial portion of the QRS complex is positive in Lead V-1. The degree of anterior rotation is not extreme since the delta wave is nearly isoelectric in Lead V-6. The an-terior rotation of the mean spatial delta wave identifies this electrocardiogram as a type A Wolff-Parkinson-White conduction abnormality (pre-excitation syndrome).

(C) The mean spatial QRS vector is orientated in the cylindrical replica of the chest. Since the QRS complex is resultantly positive in Lead V-1, the mean spatial QRS vector is flush with the frontal plane.

(D) The mean spatial T vector is rotated slightly anteriorly since the edge of the zero potential plane, which is perpendicular to the mean spatial vector, must pass through Lead V-1.

(E) Final summary figure illustrating the mean spatial QRS, ST, T, and delta wave vectors. The mean spatial delta wave vector identifies this tracing as a type A Wolff-Parkinson-White conduction abnormality (pre-excitation syndrome). Note the typical slurring of the initial portion of the QRS complex is Lead V-4 along with the short P-R interval of .1 to .13 second and QRS duration of .11 second. Warning! This type of electrocardiogram may simulate inferoposterior myocardial infarction.

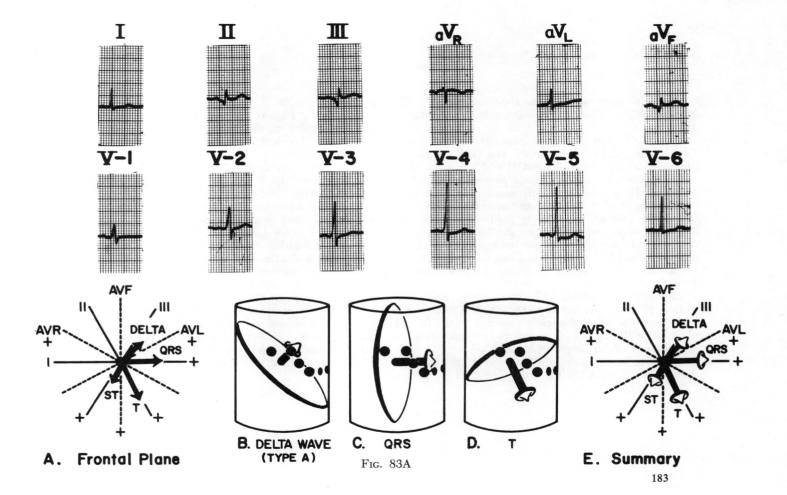

I   II   III   aV_R   aV_L   aV_F

V-1   V-2   V-3   V-4   V-5   V-6

A. Frontal Plane

B. DELTA WAVE
(TYPE A)

C. QRS

D. T

Fig. 83A

E. Summary

183

Fig. 83B. Electrocardiogram showing type B Wolff-Parkinson-White conduction abnormality (pre-excitation syndrome).

(A) The frontal plane projection of the mean spatial QRS, T, and delta wave vectors. The QRS complex is almost resultantly zero in Lead II and the mean QRS vector is illustrated as being almost perpendicular to that lead axis. (It is actually slightly negative in Lead II so it is diagrammed to project negative in that lead). The T wave is smallest and slightly positive in Lead aV$_F$. The delta wave—represented by the initial .04 portion of the QRS complex—is largest and positive in Lead aV$_L$ and small and negative in Lead II. Therefore, the mean delta wave vector is nearly perpendicular to Lead II.

(B) The mean spatial delta wave vector orientated in the cylindrical replica of the chest. The mean delta wave vector is directed slightly posterior to the frontal plane since the initial .04 portion of the QRS complex is resultantly slightly negative in Lead V-1.

(C) The mean spatial QRS vector is orientated in the cylindrical replica of the chest. The QRS complexes are almost resultantly zero in Leads V-3 and V-4. Accordingly, the edge of the zero potential plane, which is perpendicular to the mean QRS vector, must pass near them. Therefore, the mean QRS vector is rotated slightly posteriorly.

(D) The mean spatial T vector is rotated slightly anteriorly since the T wave in Lead V-1 is resultantly slightly positive.

(E) Final summary figure illustrating the mean spatial QRS, T, and delta wave vectors. Since the mean spatial delta wave vector is slightly posterior to the frontal plane rather than being anterior, the electrocardiogram is identified as being a type B Wolff-Parkinson-White conduction abnormality (pre-excitation syndrome). The mean delta wave vector is usually posteriorly directed in such tracings. Note the typical slurring of the initial QRS complex in most leads. The P-R interval is .08 to .09 second and the QRS duration is .12 second. Warning! This type of electrocardiogram can be misinterpreted as being due to inferior, or sometimes anterior, myocardial infarction.

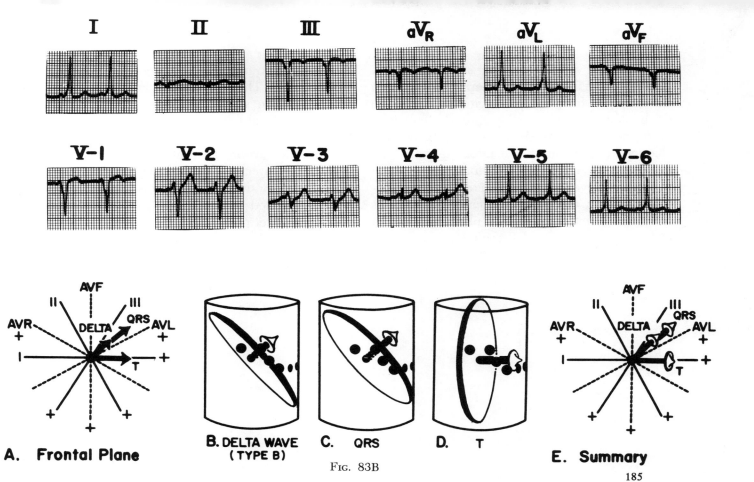

I   II   III   aV_R   aV_L   aV_F

V-1   V-2   V-3   V-4   V-5   V-6

A. **Frontal Plane**

B. **DELTA WAVE (TYPE B)**

C. **QRS**

D. **T**

E. **Summary**

F_IG. 83B

185

slurred initial vector indicating slow conduction through ordinary muscle is referred to as a *delta wave*. Other forms of pre-excitation, in which the bypass tracts presumably enter the ventricles in or near specialized conducting tissue, are characterized by short P-R intervals with little or no slurring of the initial vectors (i.e., no delta wave). However, the direction of the initial vector may deviate from normal. Many cases of paraoxysmal supraventricular tachycardia (Chapter 13) may be the result of the presence of the bypass tracts present in various forms of pre-excitation. The bypass tracts and the normal portions of the specialized conducting system presumably form two legs of reentrant loops.

When the abnormal initial vector resulting in the delta wave in the Wolff-Parkinson-White syndrome is directed anteriorly, it is called type A (fig. 83A); a delta wave vector directed posteriorly is called type B (fig. 83B). In type A, the bypass tract presumably enters the left ventricle; in type B, it enters the right ventricle.

CHAPTER SIX
Effects of Digitalis

There are several electrocardiographic effects of digitalis medication. It produces cardiac arrhythmias, prolongs conduction time, shortens electrical systole, and alters the manner of repolarization so that marked ST and T changes occur.

Although premature ventricular contraction, frequently occurring as bigeminy, is the most common cardiac arrhythmia resulting from digitalis medication, virtually any cardiac rhythm can be produced. The P-R interval is frequently prolonged because of a delay of impulse conduction at the A-V node. Occasionally the P-R interval may gradually increase during several successive heart cycles until the auricular impulse fails to be conducted through the A-V node. Under such circumstances a P wave may not be followed by a QRS complex. This type of conduction defect is called the Wenckebach phenomenon. The QRS complexes are not altered by digitalis.

In the normal subject the wave of depolarization producing the QRS complex proceeds from endocardium to epicardium and the wave of repolarization producing the T wave proceeds from epicardium to endocardium. The wave of repolarization does not follow the same path as the wave of depolarization because there is a delay of the repolarization in the subendocardial region, due, perhaps, to the altered membrane tension occurring in that area during ventricular systole. The rate and manner of cell repolarization or recovery is greatly influenced by digitalis medication. After digitalis medication, cell membrane repolarization occurs more rapidly than normally, producing a short Q-T interval. The

Q-T interval, normally over .34 second at heart rates of 75 to 95, is frequently reduced to as low as .28 second at these heart rates. The T waves may become smaller after digitalis medication; that is, the T vector becomes shorter, retaining its normal direction. This is perhaps due to some repolarization taking place from endocardium to epicardium at the same time as normal repolarization is occurring from epicardium to endocardium. Because of this, certain of the resultant instantaneous T forces are directed opposite to each other, cancelling each other, and a smaller mean T vector results. When sufficient digitalis is present, many of the subendocardial fibers recover so quickly that part of the repolarization process occurs immediately after the QRS complex and follows the same sequence as depolarization. In other words, some of the forces of repolarization occur so quickly that they are manifested during the S-T interval and since these particular forces proceed from endocardium toward the epicardium, in a manner opposite to normal, T forces are produced which are directed opposite to the QRS forces. Accordingly, a mean ST vector representing early repolariza-

tion develops following digitalization which is directed opposite to the mean QRS vector. This ST vector may become quite large, the T vector becoming smaller as the ST vector becomes larger. At times, the digitalis effect may be so marked that the entire recovery phase proceeds from endocardium to epicardium and no T waves may be found. In such a case the repolarization forces occur during the S-T interval and, when represented by a mean vector, are located roughly 180° from the mean QRS vector. As long as any T waves can be identified, the vector representing them will have the same direction that it had prior to digitalis. If digitalis is given to a patient with left ventricular hypertrophy where the mean ST and T vectors are already rotated 180° away from the mean QRS vector, little change occurs except for a shortening of the Q-T interval.

It is likely that many of the ST and T changes which accompany digitalis administration are related to changes the drug produces in the mechanism of contraction by the heart rather than entirely a direct effect on repolarization. This may explain why the electrocardiographic effects of digitalis administration vary markedly from individual to individual with the same doses and why persons with heart disease often show electrocardiographic effects to doses of digitalis which have no effect on the electrocardiogram of the normal subject. The ST and T change of digitalis effect may closely resemble the subendocardial injury of coronary insufficiency because in both instances there is a mean ST vector directed relatively opposite to the mean QRS vector and the two conditions must be differentiated on clinical grounds. An electrocardiogram may undergo little change after exercise or after digitalis alone but when digitalis has been given and the patient exercises, the ST and T changes typical of digitalis medication may occur transiently. This has practical importance since these changes are exactly the same as the ST changes encountered in the positive exercise test commonly associated with coronary insufficiency.

The electrocardiogram gives no information relative to when digitalis is needed or when the optimum effect has been reached. A patient may have evidence of clinical toxicity with nausea and vomiting and only slight changes characteristic of digitalis effect in the electrocardiogram or marked electrocardiographic effects may be present with no symptoms of clinical toxicity. In general, the need for and dosage of digitalis depends entirely on the clinical evaluation of the patient.

Figures 84, 85, 86, and 87 illustrate the effects of digitalis on the ST and T portions of the electrocardiogram.

FIG. 84. The electrocardiogram of a normal subject, 29 years of age, made prior to digitalis medication. (A) The frontal plane projection of the mean spatial QRS and T vectors. (B) The mean QRS vector is tilted 30° posteriorly because the transitional pathway passes between electrode positions V-3 and V-4. (C) The mean T vector is tilted 10° anteriorly because the transitional pathway passes through electrode position V-1. (D) Final summary figure showing the spatial arrangements of the mean QRS and T vectors. This electrocardiogram is normal.

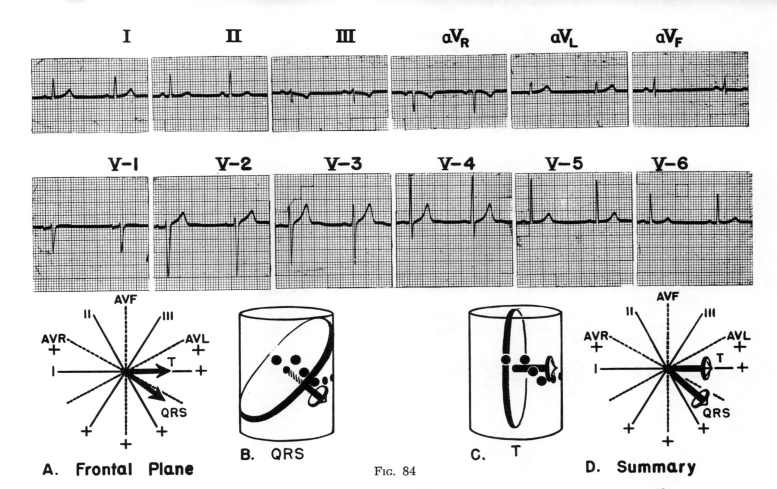

I   II   III   aV$_R$ aV$_L$ aV$_F$

V-1   V-2   V-3   V-4   V-5   V-6

A. Frontal Plane

B. QRS

C. T

D. Summary

FIG. 84

191

Fig. 85. The electrocardiogram of the same subject shown in fig. 84 made after 2 mg. of digoxin were given orally over a 24-hour period.

(A) The frontal plane projection of the mean spatial QRS and T vectors. Note that the QRS vector has not been altered by digitalis medication. The mean T vector has not changed in direction but is smaller in magnitude after digitalis medication.

(B) The mean QRS vector is tilted 30° posteriorly because the transitional pathway passes between electrode positions V-3 and V-4.

(C) The mean T vector is tilted 10° anteriorly because the transitional pathway passes through electrode position V-1.

(D) Final summary figure showing the spatial arrangement of the mean QRS and T vectors. The only significant change following digitalis medication is the decrease in magnitude of the T vector while the direction of the mean T vector remains the same. The Q-T interval has not been altered significantly in this particular instance following digitalis medication.

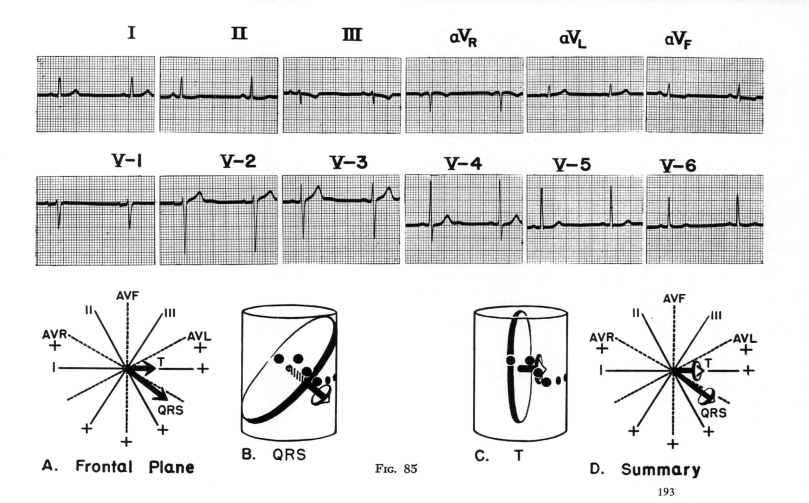

I II III aV_R aV_L aV_F

V-1 V-2 V-3 V-4 V-5 V-6

A. Frontal Plane   B. QRS   C. T   D. Summary

Fig. 85

193

Fig. 86. The electrocardiogram of a hypertensive patient, 77 years of age, made prior to digitalis medication. (A) The frontal plane projection of the mean spatial QRS and T vectors. (B) The mean QRS vector is tilted 30° posteriorly because the transitional pathway passes between electrode positions V-3 and V-4. (C) The mean T vector is tilted at least 15° anteriorly because all the precordial leads record upright T waves. (D) Final summary figure showing the spatial arrangement of the mean QRS and T vectors. This is a normal electrocardiogram.

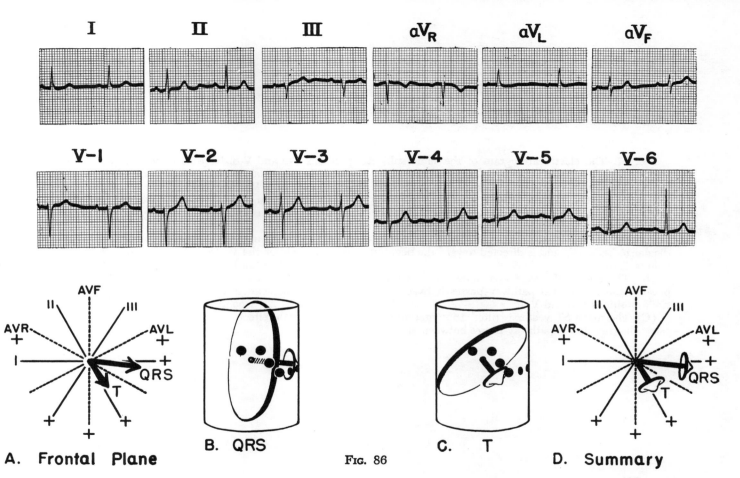

I II III aV_R aV_L aV_F

V-1 V-2 V-3 V-4 V-5 V-6

A. Frontal Plane

B. QRS

Fɪɢ. 86

C. T

D. Summary

195

FIG. 87. The electrocardiogram of the same subject shown in fig. 86 made after digitalis medication

(A) The frontal plane projection of the mean QRS, ST, and T vectors. Note that the T waves are extremely small and difficult to identify. The ST segment displacement is greatest and negative in Lead I and smallest in Lead aV_F. Accordingly, the mean ST vector is perpendicular to Lead aV_F and is directed toward the negative pole of Lead I.

(B) The mean QRS vector is tilted 30° posteriorly because the transitional pathway passes between electrode positions V-3 and V-4.

(C) The mean ST vector is tilted 15° anteriorly because the transitional pathway passes between electrode positions V-2 and V-3. Note that this will produce elevated ST segments in V-1 and V-2 and depressed ST segments in V-3, V-4, V-5, V-6.

(D) The mean T vector has not changed its position since the previous tracing, but is a great deal smaller after digitalis.

(E) Final summary figure showing the spatial arrangements of the vectors. As the T vector becomes smaller, an ST vector becomes prominent and is directed opposite to the mean QRS vector. The QT interval prior to digitalis medication was .36 second and after digitalis medication is .29 second. These findings are characteristic of digitalis effect.

196

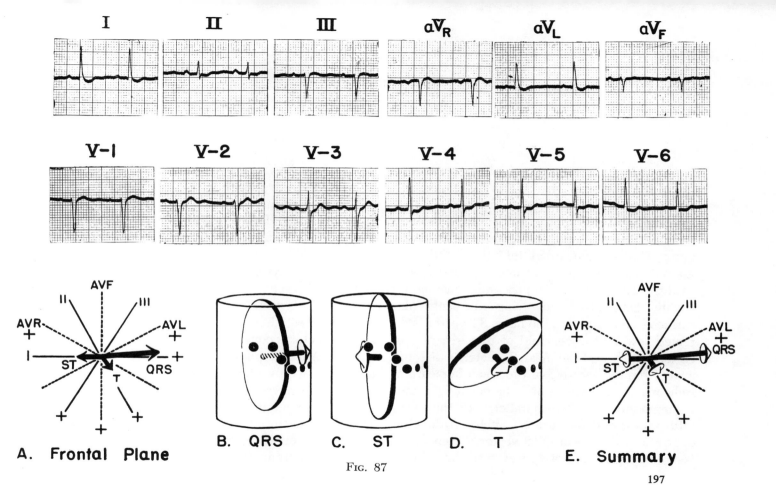

I II III aV_R aV_L aV_F

V-1 V-2 V-3 V-4 V-5 V-6

A. Frontal Plane

B. QRS

C. ST

D. T

E. Summary

Fig. 87

197

CHAPTER SEVEN

Pericarditis

The electrocardiographic findings commonly found in pericarditis are due to associated epicardial myocardial damage. Under such circumstances, epicardial injury and ischemia develop and alter the ST-T portion of the electrocardiogram. Unlike myocardial infarction, QRS abnormalities never occur in uncomplicated pericarditis. The epicardial injury and ischemia are usually generalized, involving all ventricular surfaces, and therefore the mean ST vector is directed toward the centroid of the area of epicardial injury and the mean T vector is directed away from the centroid of the area of epicardial ischemia. As a consequence, the mean ST vector is commonly relatively parallel with the mean QRS vector and the mean T vector is directed opposite to the mean QRS vector. Often the T vector change does not appear until the ST vector has largely vanished, which usually occurs in from one to two weeks.

This type of mean ST and T vector arrangement is quite different from that of ventricular hypertrophy, bundle branch block, or digitalis effect. The ST vector occasionally seen in normal subjects is always parallel with a large normally directed T vector, whereas the ST vector of pericarditis is usually associated with an oppositely directed small T vector. Also, the normal ST vector is constant from day to day, while the ST vector of pericarditis is relatively transient, lasting only a few days or weeks. Although no QRS changes occur in pericarditis, which usually differentiates it from the electrocardiogram of myocardial infarction, the two conditions may in other regards produce quite similar electrocardiograms. This is especially true when there is apical epicardial injury and ischemia resulting from coronary occlusion. Under such circumstances the mean ST vector may be directed toward the left hip and the mean T vector may be directed toward the right shoulder, resembling the vector arrangement commonly seen in pericarditis.

The electrocardiogram shown in fig. 88 illustrates the abnormal ST and T vectors commonly encountered in pericarditis.

Fɪɢ. 88. The electrocardiogram of a patient, 37 years of age, with the clinical findings of benign idiopathic pericarditis.

(A) The frontal plane projection of the mean spatial QRS, ST, and T vectors.

(B) The mean QRS vector is tilted 30° posteriorly because the transitional pathway passes between electrode positions V-3 and V-4.

(C) The mean ST vector is tilted 50° posteriorly because the transitional pathway passes between electrode positions V-4 and V-5.

(D) The mean T vector is rotated almost 80° away from the frontal plane, producing inverted T waves in all the precordial leads.

(E) Final summary figure illustrating the spatial arrangement of the vectors. The mean spatial ST vector is directed toward the centroid of diffuse epicardial injury and is nearly parallel with the mean spatial QRS vector. The mean spatial T vector is directed away from an area of diffuse epicardial ischemia. These findings are typical of pericarditis.

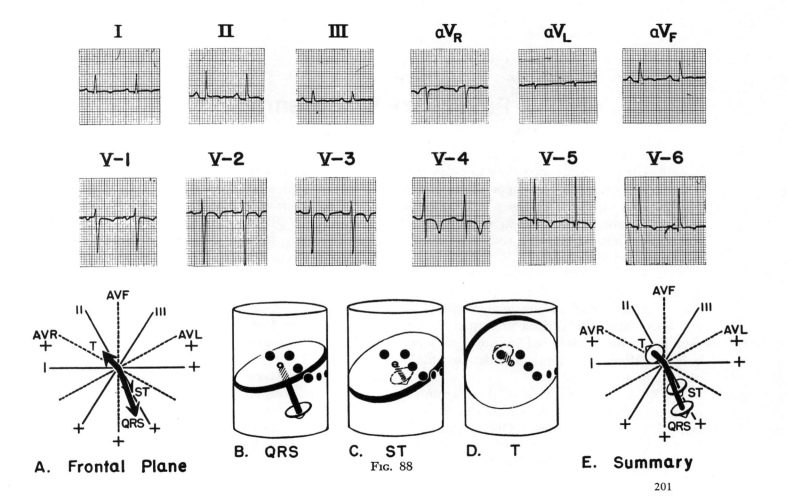

I II III aV_R aV_L aV_F

V-1 V-2 V-3 V-4 V-5 V-6

A. Frontal Plane

B. QRS

C. ST

D. T

E. Summary

Fig. 88

201

CHAPTER EIGHT

Pulmonary Embolism

Acute cor pulmonale secondary to pulmonary embolism occasionally produces electrocardiographic abnormalities. Changes in the electrocardiogram are frequently extremely transient and small pulmonary emboli produce no electrocardiographic abnormalities.

Perhaps the most common electrocardiographic finding observed after pulmonary embolism is nonspecific sinus tachycardia. It is not uncommon for various abnormal cardiac rhythms to be precipitated by pulmonary embolism, particularly auricular fibrillation or auricular tachycardia.

The QRS loop may be altered by acute cor pulmonale. This change is reflected in the electrocardiogram by a change in QRS contour. The QRS loop abnormality probably represents a type of conduction delay due to acute right ventricular dilatation. Under such circumstances the entire QRS loop shifts to the right when viewed in the frontal plane. The initial forces composing the QRS loop are directed to the left since the early forces are predominantly left ventricular forces. This may produce a Q wave in Lead III and occasionally in Lead aV_F. The terminal forces composing the QRS loop are directed to the right and anteriorly since the late forces are predominantly right ventricular forces. This produces an S wave in Lead I and R waves in Leads V-1 and V-2 which are relatively characteristic of the electrocardiogram in acute cor pulmonale. The QRS interval may be only slightly prolonged but on occasion becomes .12 second in duration and the QRS loop may resemble typical right bundle branch block. The mean QRS vector rotates to the right as a result of the altered QRS loop.

At times ST and T changes are produced by pulmonary emboli. An ST vector develops and tends to be directed toward the right shoulder away from the cardiac apex, suggesting generalized subendocardial injury of both ventricles. Frequently, the T vector becomes directed to the left and posteriorly, presumably because of right ventricular "ischemia." The latter finding may be the only abnormality or may be combined with the QRS loop abnormality. At times such a T wave abnormality may closely resemble anterior myocardial ischemia secondary to coronary occlusion.

The disturbed basic physiology responsible for the electrocardiographic abnormalities occurring after pulmonary embolism has never been completely clarified. It would seem reasonable, however, that right ventricular hypertension, dilatation, and ischemia with associated coronary insufficiency and tachycardia all play a part in producing the electrocardiographic abnormalities.

It should be recalled that clinically it is not uncommon for pulmonary embolism to precipitate myocardial infarction.

The electrocardiogram shown in fig. 89 illustrates the QRS, ST, and T abnormalities occasionally seen following pulmonary embolism.

FIG. 89. The electrocardiogram of a patient, 54 years of age, made shortly after pulmonary embolism.

(A) The frontal plane projection of the mean spatial QRS loop and ST and T vectors.

(B) The QRS loop is broken down into four successive spatial instantaneous vectors. Each of these instantaneous vectors are oriented in space producing a rough outline of the mean spatial QRS loop.

(C) The mean ST vector is rotated 40° anteriorly because the ST segment is elevated in V-1, V-2, V-3 and depressed in V-5 and V-6.

(D) The mean T vector is rotated approximately 20° posteriorly because the T wave is inverted in V-1, V-2, V-3, V-4 and upright in V-5 and V-6. Note that when the mean T vector, or any vector, is in this position, only a small amount of posterior rotation is necessary to produce inverted T waves in several of the precordial leads.

(E) Final summary figure illustrating the spatial arrangement of the vectors. The QRS loop is rotund and is inscribed in a clockwise manner. The initial forces are to the left and are rotated anteriorly, producing an initial R wave in Lead V-1. Vector four, illustrating the terminal QRS vectors, is directed to the right and anteriorly, producing an S wave in Lead I and V-2, V-3, V-4, V-5, V-6, and an R wave in V-1. The mean ST vector is directed toward the right shoulder and indicates subendocardial injury while the mean T vector is directed to the left and posteriorly indicating right ventricular ischemia. These findings are typical of acute cor pulmonale secondary to pulmonary embolism. At times only right ventricular ischemia may be present.

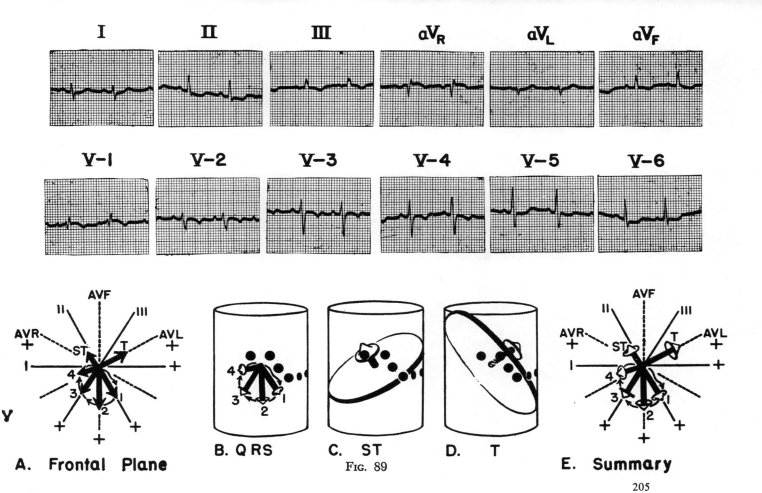

I   II   III   aV_R   aV_L   aV_F

V-1   V-2   V-3   V-4   V-5   V-6

A. Frontal Plane   B. QRS   C. ST   D. T   E. Summary

Fig. 89

205

CHAPTER NINE

Summary

The direction of the electrical forces of the heart can be determined by simple inspection of the routine electrocardiographic leads and represented by spatial vectors. The normal and abnormal electrocardiograms can be studied by such a method. In fig. 90 the spatial vector arrangements for the common electrocardiographic syndromes are illustrated.

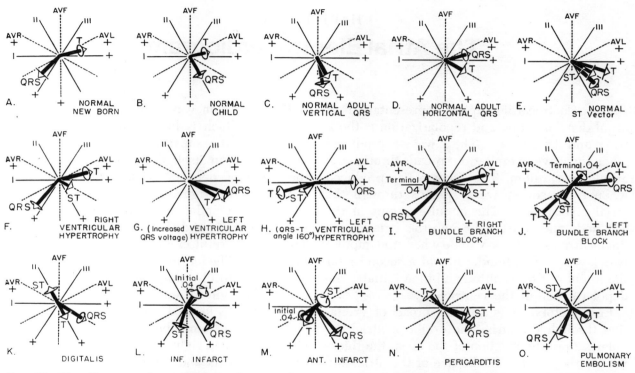

Fig. 90. The diagrams above illustrate the spatial vector arrangements for most of the electrocardiographic syndromes commonly observed in clinical practice.

CHAPTER TEN

The Atrial Electrocardiogram

The electrocardiographic representation of atrial depolarization and repolarization is the P wave and the Ta wave. The P wave is produced when the wave of excitation spreads through the atrial myocardium. The Ta wave is produced when the recovery wave spreads through the atrial myocardium. The impulse begins in the S-A node and spreads through the atria, and it finally arrives at the A-V node where the impulse is delayed. A few hundredths of a second later the impulse is transmitted and then initiates the depolarization of the ventricles.

Five factors influence the spread of excitation through the atria: the origin of atrial depolarization, the location of the atria, the thickness of the atrial wall, the size of the atria, and the loosely organized conduction pathways in the atria.

The excitation wave normally begins in the S-A node which is located in the area of the junction of the superior vena cava and right atrium. This in itself determines the direction the wave of depolarization takes. When the atrial impulse originates in some location other than the S-A node, the wave of depolarization will be changed and the P wave will be altered. This fact is useful in studying arrhythmias (see Part Two). The left atrium is not located on the left—it is centrally and posteriorly located in the chest. The right atrium is not located solely on the right—it is located anteriorly as well. These facts must be remembered as one attempts to identify left and right atrial "enlargement." The size of the atria and the thickness of the atrial wall undoubtedly influence the wave of atrial depolarization. The amount each contributes to the P wave is difficult to ascertain. There is a well-organized conduction system in the ventricles. There is no such highly developed conduction system in the atria. There are, however, at least three loosely organized and poorly developed atrial conduction pathways. These conduction pathways obviously control the path of atrial excitation to some extent. In fact, these pathways may be as important as the size and thickness of the atrial wall in determining the sequence of atrial depolarization. These pathways, which are made up of specialized cells, are influenced by the autonomic nervous system and may be altered by the size of the atrium, etc.

Atrial depolarization occurs in a sequence and produces a P loop which is vaguely reminiscent of the QRS loop which is produced in the ventricles. The instantaneous electrical forces which make up the P loop are directed anteriorly or posteriorly, inferiorly or superiorly, or to the right or left. Each of these instantaneous electrical forces influences the extremity and precordial leads and can be represented as vectors. The spatially oriented instantaneous P vectors and the mean spatial P vector can be determined by using the same technique that has been previously described on pages 3 through 42.

The Normal P Wave. The normal P wave is difficult to define and the normal range is wide. Considerable disease may be present and the P wave may remain normal. On the other hand, peculiar P waves may occur in patients without other evidence of heart disease. The height, duration, and shape of the P waves vary from subject to subject and may be different in the same subject from year to year and even minute to minute. The P wave may increase in amplitude with an increase in heart rate. (Tables are available that indicate the range of amplitude of the normal P wave in various leads for all age periods. Such tables have not proved to be too useful.) The normal P wave is usually less than 2.5 millimeters in height and less than .11 second in duration. The P wave may have a smooth contour or be slightly notched. The normal mean P vector is usually directed to the left, downward, and slightly anteriorly. It is usually located to the left of Lead axis aV_F and below Lead axis I (most frequently between $+30°$ and $+60°$) and sufficiently anterior to produce a predominately

209

upright P wave in Lead V-1 (see figs. 27 to 36). The early instantaneous P vectors are usually located to the right of and anterior to the subsequent vectors. The first portion of the P wave is produced predominately by the right atrium and the last portion of the P wave is produced predominately by the left atrium. The middle portion is produced by both atria.

Left Atrial Abnormality. The term left atrial *abnormality* is used here because we are uncertain as to the exact cause of the P wave abnormality when we suspect that the problem is located predominately in the left atrium. As implied earlier, certain P wave abnormalities may be due to interatrial conduction disturbances rather than atrial hypertrophy or atrial enlargement. Certainly the P wave may be abnormal when the left atrial pressure is normal and when there is no evidence of left atrial enlargement by x-ray examination. A left atrial abnormality *may* be reflected in the P wave of the electrocardiogram in patients with mitral stenosis, mitral regurgitation, systemic hypertension, aortic stenosis, aortic regurgitation, idiopathic hypertrophic subaortic stenosis, or left ventricular failure. Unfor-

tunately, the P wave may remain within normal limits when these diseases are present. On the other hand, a P wave abnormality may be present and the diseases mentioned may not be present. These two statements simply highlight the fact that the range of normal for the P wave overlaps the abnormal range.

Left atrial abnormality may be suspected when the P wave becomes deformed and shows certain characteristics. The P wave may become broader and larger than normal, and it may become so broad that a prominent notch may be seen at its summit. This probably results from an intra- or interatrial conduction defect. Under these circumstances the first portion of the P wave is produced primarily by depolarization of the right atrium and the last portion of the P wave is produced by depolarization of the left atrium. The notch may become so prominent in some cases of mitral stenosis that the P wave looks like the letter M (see Leads I and V-6 in fig. 40).

The P wave should be divided into two parts —the first quarter and the last three-quarters. Each of these parts can be represented by mean vectors. The first quarter vector may remain reasonably normal in patients with left atrial abnormality, since it is produced mainly by the right atrium. It is directed slightly anteriorly, to the left, and inferiorly. The last three-quarter vector may be large, directed normally or leftward in the frontal plane, and more posteriorly directed than normal when viewed in space. This should be expected, since the left atrium is truly posterior and is centrally located. The first quarter instantaneous P vectors will produce a small positive wave in Lead V-1, and the last three-quarter instantaneous P vectors will produce a large, broad negative wave in Leads V-1, V-2, and occasionally in V-3 (see Leads V-1, V-2, V-3 in fig. 40).

Right Atrial Abnormality. The term right atrial *abnormality* is used here because we are uncertain as to the exact cause of the P wave abnormality even when we suspect that the problem is located predominately in the right atrium. A right atrial abnormality *may* be reflected in the P wave of the electrocardiogram in patients with pulmonary hypertension due to mitral stenosis, primary pulmonary hypertension, left ventricu-

lar failure, pulmonary emphysema, pulmonary valve stenosis, subvalvular (infundibular) pulmonary stenosis, Ebstein's anomaly, etc. Unfortunately, the P wave may remain within normal limits when these diseases are present. On the other hand, a P wave abnormality may be present and the diseases mentioned may not be present.

Right atrial abnormality may be *suspected* when the P wave becomes deformed and shows certain characteristics. The P wave becomes tall and "peaked" (see P waves in fig. 41). Since the first portion of the P wave is produced primarily by depolarization of the right atrium, it is this portion of the P wave that becomes abnormal. After determining the *absence* of evidence of a left atrial abnormality using the criteria described above, the P wave should be divided into two parts—the first three-quarters and the last quarter. Each of these parts can be represented as mean vectors. The first three-quarter mean vector is directed inferiorly and slightly to the left—but becomes larger than normal and is directed more anteriorly than normal when there is a right atrial abnormality.

This should be expected, since the right atrium is located not only on the right but also anteriorly. The first three-quarter instantaneous P vectors will produce a large positive wave in Lead V-1, and the last one-quarter instantaneous P vectors will be normal in magnitude and direction and produce a positive wave in Lead V-1. Accordingly, the entire P wave will be large, peaked, and positive in Lead V-1 when there is a pure right atrial abnormality (see Lead V-1 in fig. 41).

Right and Left Atrial Abnormalities. Right and left atrial abnormalities may occur in the same patient and be reflected in the same electrocardiogram. This should be expected, since there are a number of diseases that can produce multiple abnormalities in the same heart. For example, mitral stenosis may produce left atrial abnormality; and when sufficient pulmonary hypertension develops, right atrial abnormality may develop.

Combined atrial abnormalities should be suspected when a few of the elements of left and right atrial abnormality are noted in the P waves of an electrocardiogram. The initial P wave

electrical forces are larger than normal and are directed inferiorly and more anteriorly than normal. This deviation from normal is produced by the right atrial abnormality. The terminal P wave electrical forces are larger than normal and are directed leftward and more posteriorly than normal. This deviation from normal is produced by the left atrial abnormality. When these electrical forces are viewed as vectors, it is simple to visualize how the first portion of the P wave in Lead V-1 would be large and positive and how the last portion of the P wave would be large and negative (see Lead V-1 in fig. 37).

A Note of Caution. Conclusions based on the analysis of P waves are often incorrect. Individuals who have correlated the P waves of the electrocardiogram with the clinical features, hemodynamic data, and autopsy findings are aware of the pitfalls that await the person who becomes rigid in his views regarding his ability to draw dogmatic conclusions from the inspection of P waves. As stated earlier, many benign conditions, such as tachycardia, autonomic nervous system stimulation, and unimportant conduction defects, may alter the P waves. Atrial myocardial infarction may produce abnormal P waves. The P waves may become abnormal in patients with valvular and myocardial disease. Many serious diseases of the heart are not associated with P wave abnormalities even when one would reason that they should be (see fig. 42). The problem is dramatically highlighted when one encounters what is thought to be a right atrial abnormality in the electrocardiogram, and it turns out that all other data suggests that there is a left atrial abnormality, or when one encounters what is thought to be a left atrial abnormality on the electrocardiogram and all other data suggests that there is a right atrial abnormality.

The P-R Interval. The P-R interval is determined by identifying the time that elapses from the beginning of the P wave to the beginning of the QRS complex. The P-R interval represents the time required for atrial depolarization plus the delay of the impulse in the A-V node and conducting system. The length of the P-R interval varies with age and heart rate (see Table 1 in Appendix). In the adult, the upper limit of normal is .20 second. First-degree atrioventricu-

lar block is said to exist when the P-R interval is longer than normal (see Chapter 17). First-degree A-V block may develop as a result of digitalis medication, rheumatic fever, coronary atherosclerosis, other types of heart disease, and infectious diseases such as mumps and diphtheria.

The Atrial T Wave. When the wave of depolarization spreads through the atrial myocardium it produces the P wave in the electrocardiogram. The electrical forces associated with the wave of depolarization can be represented as a mean vector. A mean vector representing all the instantaneous P vectors is normally directed (1) inferiorly, (2) leftward, and (3) slightly anteriorly, flush with the frontal plane or slightly posterior. The wave of *repolarization* spreads through the atrial myocardium and produces a "T wave"—the Ta wave. *A mean vector representing all the instantaneous atrial repolarization vectors is directed opposite to the mean P vector. This is different from the normal mean ventricular T vector which is directed relatively parallel to the mean QRS vector. This* difference may occur because the transmyocardial pressure gradient is different in the atria as compared with the ventricles. The atrial T wave is very small and frequently cannot be identified on the clinical electrocardiogram. The initial instantaneous atrial T wave vectors are written almost immediately after the initial instantaneous P vectors. Therefore, a significant portion of the wave of repolarization is written during the wave of atrial depolarization (P wave). The Ta wave continues, however, through the P-R interval. Occasionally a portion of the atrial T wave can be identified just after the P wave (see Lead V-2 in fig. 32 and Lead V-6 in fig. 40). A portion of the atrial T wave may sometimes be seen just after the QRS complex and is one of the many causes of a displaced S-T segment. This is likely to occur when the P and Ta waves are large and the heart rate is rapid. The atrial T waves may be seen more easily in tracings showing A-V block.

PART TWO

The Cardiac Arrhythmias

CHAPTER ELEVEN
Introduction to Arrhythmias

Abnormalities of cardiac rhythm and conduction are common. They may be discovered either subjectively by the patient or during a physical examination by the physician, or they may go unnoticed. In any event, the diagnosis of the exact nature of the rhythm disturbance almost always is dependent upon the electrocardiogram. A rational approach to the accurate electrocardiographic analysis of cardiac rhythms requires (1) knowledge of the physiology of cardiac impulse formation and conduction (fig. 91), (2) proper selection and length of the electrocardiographic leads to be studied, and (3) an organized system of analysis.

Physiology of Cardiac Impulse Formation and Conduction. The two physiologic properties of the heart of primary importance in rhythm disturbances are *automaticity* and *conduction*.

Automaticity is the physiological term denoting the process of impulse formation. It also implies "rate" of impulse formation. Automaticity is a function of the highly specialized pacemaker cells. Most electrically active cells maintain a steady charge across their cell membranes when they are in the resting state. This charge is called the "resting transmembrane potential." The potential does not change until an impulse arrives and lowers the membrane potential to a level known as the "threshold potential." When the threshold potential is reached, the cell membrane rapidly and completely depolarizes. After this, the cell repolarizes to the original resting potential. The charge remains steady until the arrival of the next impulse. However, the *pacemaker cells* of the heart possess some unique features. Instead of remaining at a steady rest-

217

ing transmembrane potential following repolarization, they *spontaneously* discharge slowly until the threshold potential is reached, at which point complete, rapid depolarization occurs. Thus, the most significant difference between the pacemaker cell and ordinary electrically active cells is the ability of the pacemaker cell to undergo spontaneous depolarization, allowing impulses to be formed de novo. Once formed, these impulses can be conducted through the rest of the heart. Any influence which (1) changes the transmembrane potential at the end of repolarization, (2) changes the threshold potential, or (3) changes the rate of the slow, spontaneous depolarization phase will change the frequency of depolarization of the automatic cells. In addition, the pacemaker cells in the various areas of the heart have markedly different inherent rates of impulse formation (see fig. 91).

The automatic pacemaker cells in the sinus node, which normally initiate the cardiac electrical impulse, have a physiologic periodicity of 60 to 100 impulses per minute. The automatic cells at the A-V junctional level (i.e., the atrial margin of the A-V node, portions of the A-V node itself, and the bundle of His) have a periodicity of 40 to 60 impulses per minute, while those at the ventricular level have an inherent rate of 20 to 40 impulses per minute. This arrangement of decreasing inherent rate of lower levels allows the next lower level to assume pacemaker function should a higher center fail, but prevents the lower centers from usurping pacemaker function under physiologic conditions. Several cell types which ordinarily do not manifest automaticity under normal conditions become automatic as a result of pharmacologic or pathologic influences.

Conduction is the term denoting the ability to propagate the formed impulse throughout the heart. This property permits the conduction system to rapidly propagate an impulse to all parts of the myocardium in an orderly physiologic sequence. Conduction may be altered or blocked (1) by physiologic stimuli, (2) by a number of pathologic states, and (3) by pharmacologic agents.

The Sequence of Cardiac Excitation. The cardiac electrical impulse is normally initiated in the automatic cells of the sinus node (fig. 91). The impulse then passes into the surrounding atrial tissue and is conducted through the atria to the A-V node. The impulse passes through the A-V node and the common bundle of His to the left and right bundle branches (fig. 91). The impulse is then conducted to the left and right ventricular muscle cells through the ramifications of the Purkinje network.

General Mechanisms of Arrhythmias. Arrhyth-

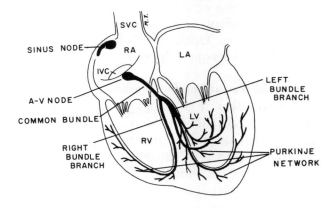

Fig. 91. The impulse-forming and -conducting system of the heart. The cardiac impulse is normally formed in the *sinus node*, located at the junction between the superior vena cava (SVC) and the right artium (RA). From the site of impulse formation, the impulse enters the right atrial tissue (across the so-called S-A junction, which probably is no more than a physiological junction whose existence becomes apparent only in disease states) and courses through the right atrium toward the *A-V*

node and to the left atrium (LA). The passage of the impulse is delayed at the A-V node and after this delay passes into the *common bundle* (the bundle of His). The impulse then moves into the *left bundle branch* and the *right bundle branch*. Depolarization of the septum, with the wave of depolarization moving from left to right, occurs while the impulse continues to be propagated through the distal ramifications of the two bundle branches. The impulse continues into the intramyocardial conduction system, the *Pukinje network*. The wave of myocardial depolarization spreads through the apex of the heart and then up the free walls of the right ventricle (RV) and the left ventricle (LV). Finally, the wave spreads around to the posterior basal portion of the heart.

The normal rate of impulse formation in the sinus node is 60 to 100 impulses per minute. Under some circumstances, however, it may form impulses much more rapidly or more slowly. Pacemaker activity is also present in other areas of the heart and may take over either (1) by increasing their rate of impulse formation *above* that of the sinus node cells or (2) by the sinus node cells decreasing their rate of impulse formation *below* that of the other sites of impulse formation. Cells in the area of the A-V node have pacemaker function and normally form impulses at the rate of 40 to 60 per minute. Pacemaker cells in the ventricles normally form impulses at the rate of 20 to 40 per minute. The descending inherent rate of impulse formation at the lower levels provides a safety mechanism whereby a lower center may pace the heart if the higher centers fail; but the lower centers will not take over the pacemaker function unnecessarily, since their inherent rate is slower than that of the higher pacemaker.

mias may be attributable to disorders of automaticity, disorders of conduction, or a combination of both. Automaticity may be either *increased* or *decreased*. Abnormal conduction generally means a *decreased* conductivity, but rarely rhythm disturbances may result from impulses during the phase of *supernormal conduction*.

Any stimulus which causes the automatic cells in any location to increase their rate of impulse formation is said to have increased the automaticity of these cells. For instance, increased automaticity of the cells of the sinus node results in sinus tachycardia and increased automaticity of a pacemaker focus in the ventricle may result in a form of ventricular tachycardia.

Electrocardiographic Lead Selection and Length of Tracing. The analysis of most arrhythmias and conduction disturbances requires the recognition of the relationship between P waves and the QRS complexes, and a lead which records both clearly is often essential. Usually standard Lead II or Lead V-1 will suffice. However, even in these leads, the P waves may be small or obscured by QRS complexes or by T waves. Therefore, special techniques may be required to demonstrate P waves. Such techniques may include an exploratory chest electrode, an esophageal electrode, or a transvenous right atrial electrode.

In most instances, a length of electrocardiographic tracing equivalent to 15 or 30 seconds will be sufficient to analyze the events of the cardiac rhythm. Occasionally, however, tracings of 60 to 120 seconds duration or more will be necessary.

General Versus Specific Diagnoses. In an emergency situation, it is often necessary to make a quick general diagnosis of the rhythm disturbance (such as differentiating between supraventricular and ventricular tachycardia), rather than attempt to elucidate the specific mechanisms involved. The rapid initiation of appropriate therapy in such cases may be lifesaving. Under other circumstances, however, it is desirable to develop the habit of attempting to define the precise mechanism of each abnormal rhythm, using a standard and orderly approach. These habits, fully developed, will assist in making the rapid general diagnosis in the emergency situation much easier and more accurate.

CHAPTER TWELVE

The A-V Diagram

The more obvious arrhythmias are easily and accurately identified by pattern recognition. However, this method of analysis lacks the precision and order of a systematic approach and makes the diagnosis of more complex arrhythmias difficult or impossible.

The A-V Diagram. (This is also called A-V ladder, laddergram, or Lewis lines.) The A-V diagram was devised to demonstrate graphically the sequence of events in an arrhythmia. It is a simple and precise method of depicting the time relationships of cardiac electrical events.

The only direct rhythm information available from the electrocardiogram is the occurrence of atrial muscular depolarization (P wave) and ventricular muscular depolarization (QRS complex). All else is inferred from the relationships between the P waves, the QRS complexes, and the P-R intervals. Thus, the need for an orderly approach to study these relationships is obvious. The A-V diagram, properly used, can provide the necessary method.

The A-V diagram (fig. 92) is mounted (or drawn) below the electrocardiogram to be analyzed. The A level represents atrial depolarization (P waves), and the V level represents ventricular depolarization (QRS complexes). The A-V level is used to represent conduction, and sometimes impulse formation, in the A-V conduction system, or junction, i.e., in the conduction pathway between the atria and the ventricles.

Rate. All intervals—P-P, R-R, P-R, and others when necessary—are carefully measured and noted on the diagram. When measuring intervals, always measure from the *beginning* of one

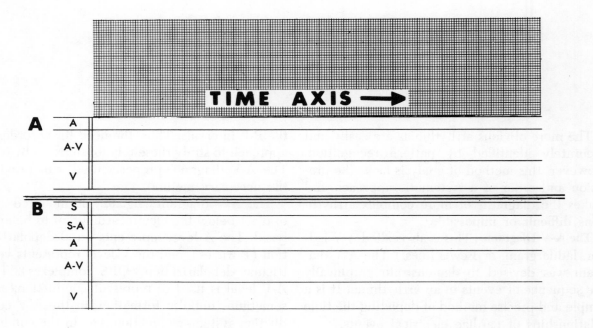

FIG. 92. (A) The usual A-V diagram for analysis of arrhythmias. The A level of the diagram is used to represent atrial depolarization (the P wave); the V level is used to demonstrate ventricular depolarization (the QRS complex); and the A-V level is used to analyze and represent A-V conduction. (B) Diagram used in the special situation where an abnormality of sinoatrial conduc-tion (i.e., conduction from the site of impulse formation in the sinus node to the atrial musculature) is suspected. In addition to the standard A, V, and A-V levels, an S level for sinus impulse formation and an S-A level for conduction from the site of impulse formation to the atrial musculature are included.

event to the *beginning* of the next, e.g., from the beginning of one P wave to the beginning of the next or from the beginning of the P wave to the beginning of the QRS complex. Measurements are best made with a pair of fine-point calipers, several types of which are available commercially.

It is useful to remember the rate-interval relationships for the more common intervals (fig. 93). An interval of .20 second occurs when the rate is 300 per minute, .40 second equals 150 per minute, .60 second equals 100 per minute, and 1.00 second equals 60 per minute.

The A Level. The P waves should be first identified on the electrocardiogram, if possible, and

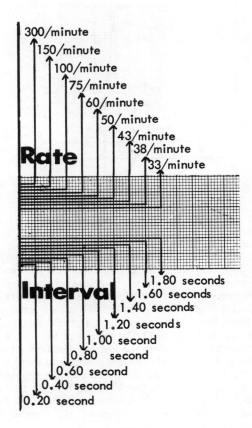

FIG. 93. Rate-interval relationship. When the rate of a cardiac event is 300 times per minute, the interval of time occurring between the events is .20 second or one large square on the ECG paper. When the event is occuring 150 times per minute, the interval is .40 second or two large squares. The diagram demonstrates some of the rate-interval relationships in the more common range. A table giving more complete rate-interval information is in the Appendix. Just as the horizontal axis from left to right indicates time on the electrocardiogram, it also indicates time on the A-V diagram.

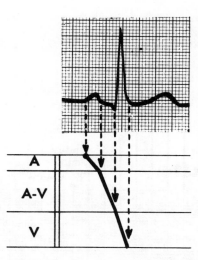

Fig. 94. Representation of a normal P-QRS complex on the A-V diagram. The beginning of the P wave is represented on the top line of the *A* level of the diagram, and the end of the P wave is noted on the line between the *A* and *A-V* levels. The two points are connected, giving a sloped line which represents both the direction and duration of the P wave. The beginning of the QRS complex is noted as a point on the line between the *AV* and *V* levels, and the end of the QRS is noted on the bottom line of the *V* level. Again, the two points are connected, giving a sloping line in the *V* level. Finally, the end point of the P wave and the beginning point of the QRS complex are connected to represent the normal A-V conduction.

represented in the *A* level of the diagram. Since atrial depolarization is not an instantaneous event (the P wave has a measurable duration) and since the horizontal axis of the diagram indicates time, P wave duration is indicated by sloping the P wave representation on the diagram so as to indicate time. If the atrial impulse is normally conducted from the sinus node to the A-V node (anterograde conduction) and is therefore upright in standard Lead II, the slope representing atrial depolarization time is directed from above downward (fig. 94). If atrial depolarization occurs retrograde from the A-V node or ventricle backward (P wave inverted in Lead II), the slope is drawn from below upward along the time axis (fig. 95). Atrial *fusion beats* occur when the timing between an anterograde impulse and a retrograde impulse, or between two different atrial impulses, is such that each depolarizes part of the atrial myocardium. They are represented by the anterograde and retrograde lines meeting in the middle of the *A* level (fig. 95).

The V Level. After the P waves have been represented on the *A* level of the diagram—or be-

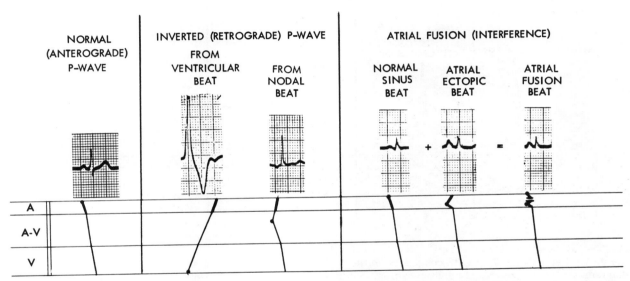

FIG. 95. Representation of P wave on the A-V diagram. (All complexes from Lead II and impulse origins represented by dots.) The first complex is normal and shows normal P wave representation. The second and third complexes show retrograde P waves (conducted through the atria from an impulse originating below them). The slope of the line is now from the bottom of the A level to the top along the time axis, indicating clearly that the impulse which depolarizes the atria came from below. The last three complexes demonstrate atrial fusion. When two sites of impulse formation can each function independently of each other, each may depolarize part of the atria when the timing is correct, and a P wave intermediate between the two independent forms results. This is represented as shown in the last complex.

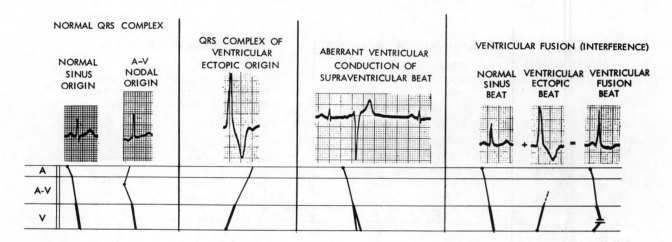

FIG. 96. Representation of QRS complexes on the A-V diagram. All complexes resulting from normal conduction of supraventricular impulses, whatever the site of impulse formation (sinus, ectopic atrial, or nodal), are represented by the normal QRS notation as demonstrated in the first two complexes. If, however, a beat of supraventricular origin is conducted through the ventricles along an aberrant pathway of conduction, the A-V diagram notation is as shown in the fourth complex. A beat of ectopic ventricular origin is represented by noting the *beginning* of the QRS complex at the *bottom* of the V level and the *end* at the *top*, as shown in the third complex. Finally, fusion beats at the ventricular level are approached and represented by essentially the same technique as at the atrial level, as shown by the last three complexes on the illustration.

226

fore this if the P waves are obscure and difficult to identify—the QRS complexes are represented on the V level of the diagram. The same rules determine the representation of time and the site of impulse origin. Fig. 94 demonstrates the QRS representation of a normally conducted ventricular impulse. Fig. 96 demonstrates the proper method to indicate the QRS complex on the A-V diagram for a nodal beat, a ventricular beat, aberrant ventricular conduction, and ventricular fusion beats.

The A-V Level. After all identifiable P waves and QRS complexes have been represented on the diagram, A-V conduction is represented. The distal end of the P wave line is connected to the proximal end of the QRS line. The A-V line slope thus indicates A-V conduction duration (fig. 94). Fig. 97 demonstrates the method of representing various types of events in the A-V junction. A-V block with a dropped beat (for example, 2:1 A-V block in which only one of every two atrial impulses can be conducted through the conduction system to discharge the ventricular myocardium) is represented by a line extending partway down the A-V level (fig. 97). Anterograde and retrograde conduction of an impulse formed in the A-V junction tissue is represented as shown in fig. 97.

Interference, which occurs when two impulses approach each other from different directions and thus prevent each other's passage, is also demonstrated in fig. 97.

The use of the A-V diagram in diagramming specific abnormalities of impulse formation and/or conduction will be presented in more detail later. Fig. 98 demonstrates the sequences used in the construction of the complete diagram, using a normal sinus rhythm as an example.

Fig. 97. Representation of events in the A-V junction on the A-V diagram. When an impulse originates in the A-V junction, conduction may occur anterograde to the ventricles and retrograde to the atria. An arbitrary point is chosen on the A-V diagram time axis to indicate the time of impulse formation, and this point must precede any of the electrical events of the complex (P wave and QRS complex). Then the retrograde P wave, if present, and the anterograde QRS complex are noted in the standard manner. The representation is completed as shown in the first complex. The phenomenon of interference between two impulses coming at each other from different directions in the A-V junction (and thus blocking each other's passage) is represented in the second and third complexes. In essence, this phenomenon is the same as fusion beats, but since it is occurring in the A-V junction, there is no direct electrocardiographic representation of it other than physiological block of further conduction of both impulses. Pathological block representation is shown in the last two sequences of complexes in the figure. The first group of complexes is from a tracing showing 2:1 A-V block, and the second group is from a case of complete heart block.

A-V DIAGRAM NOTATIONS OF A-V CONDUCTION

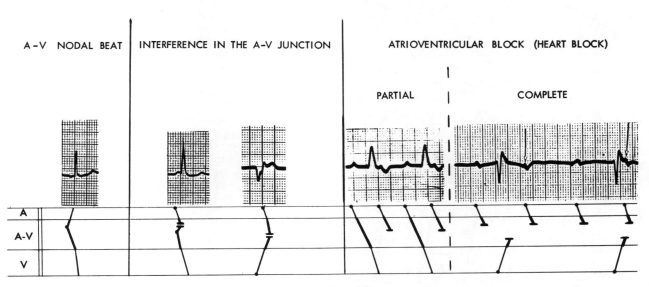

A-V NODAL BEAT	INTERFERENCE IN THE A-V JUNCTION	ATRIOVENTRICULAR BLOCK (HEART BLOCK)

FIG. 97

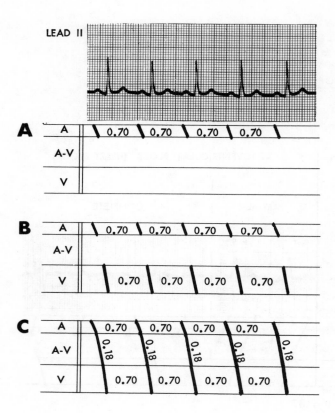

LEAD II

A	A	\ 0.70 \ 0.70 \ 0.70 \ 0.70 \
	A-V	
	V	

B	A	\ 0.70 \ 0.70 \ 0.70 \ 0.70 \
	A-V	
	V	\ 0.70 \ 0.70 \ 0.70 \ 0.70 \

C	A	\ 0.70 \ 0.70 \ 0.70 \ 0.70 \
	A-V	0.18 0.18 0.18 0.18 0.18
	V	\ 0.70 \ 0.70 \ 0.70 \ 0.70 \

Fig. 98. An electrocardiogram showing normal sinus rhythm demonstrates the sequence of steps in the construction of an A-V diagram. (A) The diagram is mounted or drawn below the electrocardiogram and the P waves identified and represented at the A level. The P-P intervals are measured and recorded. (B) The QRS complexes are identified and represented at the V level. The R-R intervals are measured and recorded. Intervals are measured from the *beginning* of one QRS complex to the *beginning* of the next. The same rule applies to the P-P intervals. (C) The final step is the representation of A-V conduction at the A-V level. This step is often the most difficult, and frequently the most important, and will be discussed later in more detail.

230

CHAPTER THIRTEEN

Variations in Sinus Node Rhythms and Atrial Arrhythmias

Sinus Arrhythmia and Wandering Pacemaker. Not all variations of sinus node impulse formation are abnormal, and two common mechanisms which fall into the category of normal variants are sinus arrhythmia and wandering pacemaker.

Sinus arrhythmia is common in childhood and tends to disappear with advancing age, but may also be seen in normal adults. It is often, but not always, related to the respiratory cycle. Characteristic of sinus arrhythmia is a normal sinus pacemaker which alternately slows and speeds up. Normal atrial depolarization pattern (i.e., normal P waves), normal A-V conduction (i.e., normal P-R interval), and normal QRS configuration are present. This arrhythmia involves only the rate of impulse formation by cells of the sinus node. Thus, the P-P and R-R intervals are equally affected in each cycle and of equal duration in any given cycle (fig. 99). The minimal variation in cycle length between the shortest cycle and the longest cycle in a sinus arrhythmia is .12 second.

A wandering pacemaker within the sinus node (fig. 100) is characterized electrocardiographically by rate changes as seen in ordinary sinus arrhythmia plus P wave variations and minor P-R interval changes with rate. The P waves tend to be taller and P-R intervals longer with a faster rate. It also may be *phasic* (i.e., related to the respiratory cycle) or *nonphasic*. A wandering pacemaker within the S-A node does not, in itself, indicate disease. *A wandering atrial pacemaker* (wandering between the sinus node

231

and A-V node) can be diagnosed when the rate changes of sinus arrhythmia are associated with more marked P wave and P-R interval variations (such as biphasic or inverted P waves in Lead II). The P waves which are intermediate between the upright sinus node beats and the inverted retrograde A-V nodal P waves are usually atrial fusion beats. (See Chapter 18.)

Sinus Bradycardia. Sinus bradycardia is defined as a heart rate of less than 60 beats per minute with a normal sinus mechanism. It is a normal variant in well-conditioned athletes at rest, and in normal sleep in healthy individuals. It may also be caused by increased parasympathetic tone of any etiology and may occur in acute inferior myocardial infarction. The electrocardiographic findings include a normal P wave, normal QRS configuration, and a normal P-R inter-

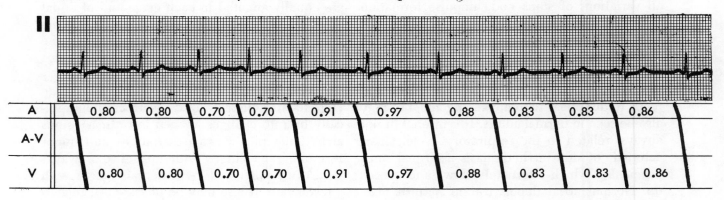

II										
A	0.80	0.80	0.70	0.70	0.91	0.97	0.88	0.83	0.83	0.86
A-V										
V	0.80	0.80	0.70	0.70	0.91	0.97	0.88	0.83	0.83	0.86

Fig. 99. Sinus arrhythmia. There is a normal sinus node mechanism of impulse formation, normal conduction, and a normal ventricular response. There is a variation in the rate of sinus node impulse formation which is greater than .12 second between the longest and short-est cycles (longest cycle = .97 second, shortest cycle = .70 second; therefore, variation = .27 second). The lack of variation in P wave morphology and in P-R interval differentiates sinus arrhythmia from a wandering pacemaker.

232

val with a P-P and R-R interval of greater than 1.00 second (fig. 101).

Sinus Tachycardia. Sinus tachycardia is defined as a heart rate greater than 100 beats per minute, with a normal sinus mechanism of impulse formation. It occurs frequently in both cardiac and noncardiac disease states, as well as in normal adaptive physiologic responses to exercise, fright, or other sympathetic stimuli. Rapid sinus tachycardia in adults usually does not exceed 150 to 160 beats per minute, although it occasionally occurs with rates as fast as 170 to 180 per minute. Further, in a few individuals, it may reach or exceed 200 per minute under conditions of extreme exercise. In young children, on the other hand, sinus tachycardia not uncommonly may exceed 200 beats per minute. With slower rates of sinus tachycardia, normal P waves and normal QRS complex duration and configuration, and normal P-R intervals, are the rule and are easily recognized (fig. 102). However, when the rate increases to the point where the P waves may be buried in the preceding T waves and the rate approaches that seen in ectopic tachycardias (e.g., paroxysmal atrial tachycardia), the recognition of sinus tachycardia becomes more difficult (fig. 103). In this latter situation, diagnostic clues favoring sinus tachycardia include gradual slowing of the rate over a period of minutes to hours and the response to carotid sinus pressure (slowing, followed by a gradual return to the original rate in a few seconds to a minute). These points will be discussed further in the section on the differential diagnosis of tachycardias.

Paroxysmal Atrial Tachycardia. Paroxysmal atrial tachycardia denotes an abnormal rhythm in which a rapid ectopic focus in the atrium has become the pacemaker of the heart. The heart rate is in the range of 140 to 240 (usually 170 to 220 beats per minute). It is frequent in normal younger people, more commonly in the female, and in patients with the Wolff-Parkinson-White syndrome. There is almost always 1:1 conduction of the ectopic atrial impulses, producing a ventricular rate equal to the ectopic atrial rate. When an ectopic atrial tachycardia is accompanied by heart block (such as 2:1, 3:1, or higher or variable block), the implication is that there is a relative or absolute abnormality of

233

Fig. 100. Wandering pacemaker. There is a rhythmic slowing and speeding of the heart rate as in sinus arrhythmia. However, the P waves tend to be taller and the P-R intervals slightly longer when the P-P interval shortens (i.e., when the heart rate increases). Conversely, the P waves are shorter and the P-R intervals shorter when the heart rate decreases. This is characteristic of so-called *wandering pacemaker within the sinus node*. If the shortening of the P waves in Lead II progresses to the point of inversion of the P waves, a *wandering atrial pacemaker* would be diagnosed (i.e., wandering to the A-V node). Inversion of the P-wave in Lead III alone does not have the same significance since this may occur from respiratory influences alone—in the absence of a wandering pacemaker.

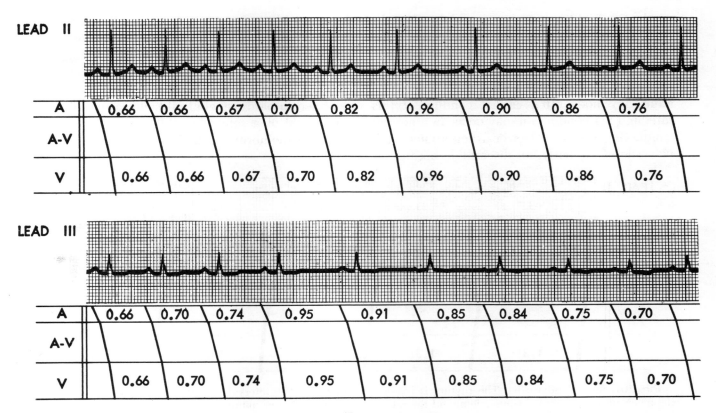

FIG. 100

conduction, which may be caused by digitalis or by disease of the A-V conduction system. The exception to this is the unusual case of paroxysmal atrial tachycardia in which the ectopic atrial rate exceeds 220 to 250 per minute. The normal adult A-V node often cannot conduct at this rate, and 2:1 conduction may occur in a normal conducting system. Electrocardiographically, P waves are frequently not discernible because of the rapid rate (fig. 104). Occasionally, a low atrial ectopic focus may produce a slow paroxysmal atrial tachycardia with a rate in the range of 120 or so per minute, in which the P waves are readily identifiable. When the P waves are identified in paroxysmal atrial tachycardia, they are usually of a somewhat different configuration from the normal sinus P waves of the same patient.

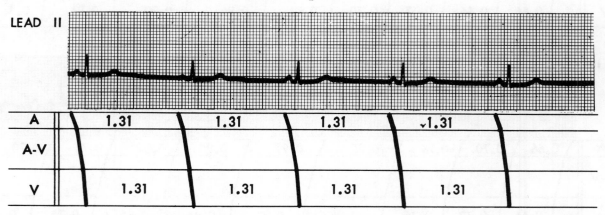

FIG. 101. Sinus bradycardia. The rhythm is regular, the mechanism is of normal sinus origin, and the rate is less than 60 per minute. In this tracing the P-P and R-R intervals are 1.31 seconds; the rate therefore is 46 per minute. An R-R interval of 1.00 second represents a rate of exactly 60 per minute; thus an interval greater than 1.00 second indicates a rate of less than 60 per minute.

Atrial Flutter. Although atrial flutter is generally categorized as a regular arrhythmia (such as sinus tachycardia or paroxysmal atrial tachycardia) becuse of its effect on atrial and ventricular electrocardiographic events, it is more closely related pathophysiologically to the irregular group of arrhythmias (such as atrial fibrillation). The precise mechanism of atrial flutter remains controversial, but it is probably not due to a discrete focus in the atrium. A circus move-

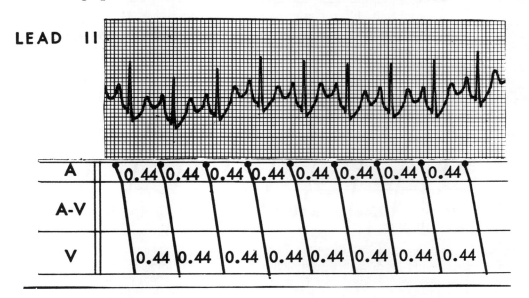

Fig. 102. Sinus tachycardia. The P-P and R-R intervals are .44 second, indicating a heart rate of 136 per minute. The P-R intervals are normal, indicating normal conduction from atria to ventricles. Thus, this tracing demonstrates a moderate sinus tachycardia.

237

ment or multiple reentry mechanism seems likely.

The *atrial rate* in atrial flutter is usually between 250 and 350 per minute and commonly

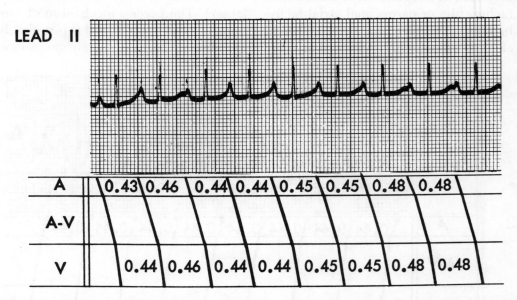

LEAD II

A	0.43	0.46	0.44	0.44	0.45	0.45	0.48	0.48
A-V								
V	0.44	0.46	0.44	0.44	0.45	0.45	0.48	0.48

Fig. 103. Sinus tachycardia. The fourth, fifth, sixth, and seventh P waves would be difficult to distinguish from the T waves of the preceding beats were it not for the slight variation in heart rate which separates the P waves from the T waves in the first, third, eighth, and ninth complexes. P waves are not ordinarily obscured by T waves at this rate (133 per minute); however, the first-degree heart block (prolonged P-R interval) in this case is responsible for the obscured P waves. Slight rhythmic variation in the rate of a supraventricular tachycardia tends to favor the diagnosis of sinus tachycardia, rather than paroxysmal atrial tachycardia or atrial flutter. The rate variation in atrial fibrillation is uusally erratic, rather than rhythmic.

238

approximates 300 per minute. Since even a normal A-V node can rarely conduct at this rate and atrial flutter is most frequently associated with organic disease, flutter is almost always accompanied by some degree of A-V conduction disturbance, such as 2:1 conduction. Thus, the *rate of ventricular response* in atrial flutter does not often exceed 150 to 160 beats per minute. In fact, any time a rate of 150 per minute is seen, atrial flutter with 2:1 conduction should be considered unless P waves are easily identifiable. Since the rate of flutter tends to remain relatively constant and the degree of A-V block varies from time to time, the ventricular rate in this arrhythmia may vary erratically between 150 (2:1 conduction), 100 (3:1 conduction), and 75 (4:1 conduction); or, on the other hand, it may remain constant at 150, 100, or 75 per minute.

The diagnosis is very simple when typical sawtooth flutter waves and a high degree of A-V block are present (fig. 105). However, when the ventricular rate is rapid (fig. 106) or the flutter waves atypical, differentiation from other tachycardias may be difficult. Carotid sinus

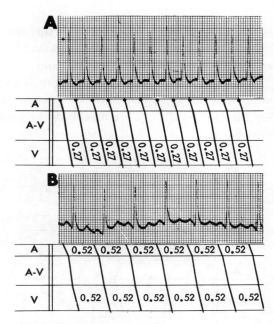

Fig. 104. Paroxysmal atrial tachycardia. (A) A short strip obtained during an attack of paroxysmal atrial tachycardia, demonstrating a heart rate of 222 beats per minute (R-R interval = .27 second). The P waves cannot be discerned because of the extremely rapid rate. (B) After abrupt conversion to a normal sinus mechanism, the heart rate is 115 beats per minute (R-R interval = .52 second). The P waves are now easily seen.

239

pressure, when effective, may help in this situation, since it increases the degree of A-V block, decreasing the ventricular response and allowing the flutter waves to become obvious. Occasionally, carotid sinus pressure speeds up the flutter rate or rarely even converts it to atrial fibrillation.

Atrial Fibrillation. As in the case of atrial flutter, the precise mechanism responsible for atrial fibrillation remains obscure. Several theories have been proposed, but none has been conclusively proved. Among the causes of atrial fibrillation are coronary artery disease, mitral valve disease, and thyrotoxicosis.

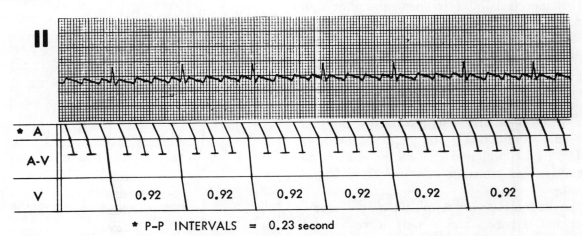

FIG. 105. Atrial flutter with 4:1 A-V conduction. Typical sawtooth flutter waves and the high degree of A-V block with consequent paucity of QRS complexes make the flutter pattern simple to recognize. The atrial flutter rate is 260 per minute (P-P interval = .23 second) and the ventricular rate is 65 per minute (R-R interval = .92 second). Only one of each four flutter waves is conducted through the A-V junction to depolarize the ventricles—hence the term 4:1 A-V conduction.

240

Electrocardiographically, atrial activity in atrial fibrillation is represented by irregular waves, which may be coarse or fine, at a rate which is often well over 400 per minute. Some-times the fibrillatory waves may be so fine as to be unrecognizable on the clinical electrocardiogram. In this situation, only the QRS-T complex appears on the electrocardiogram, without obvi-

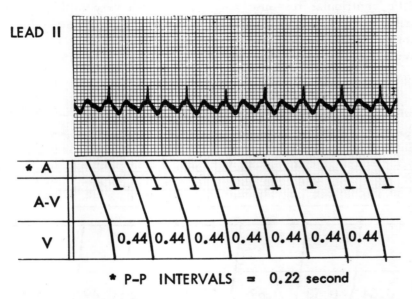

LEAD II

* A

A-V

V 0.44 | 0.44 | 0.44 | 0.44 | 0.44 | 0.44 | 0.44

* P-P INTERVALS = 0.22 second

FIG. 106. Atrial flutter with 2:1 A-V conduction. The atrial flutter rate is 272 per minute (P-P interval = .22 second), and the ventricular rate is 136 per minute (R-R interval = .44 second). Sawtooth flutter waves may be less obvious in the presence of the more rapid ventricular response. As the atrial flutter rate increases and/or the ventricular response increases, atrial flutter becomes more difficult to recognize.

241

ous atrial activity. At the other extreme, the fibrillatory waves may be extremely coarse and relatively regular, resembling atrial flutter waves.

The characteristic ventricular response pattern in atrial fibrillation is a grossly irregular rhythm with a normal QRS duration and contour (fig. 107). With digitalis intoxication and/or disease of the A-V conducting system, the ventricular response in atrial fibrillation may be regular (fig. 108) because of a high-grade A-V block and a nodal pacemaker. On the other hand, with very rapid ventricular response in atrial fibrillation, the rhythm may appear to be regular.

The ventricular rate in untreated atrial fibril-

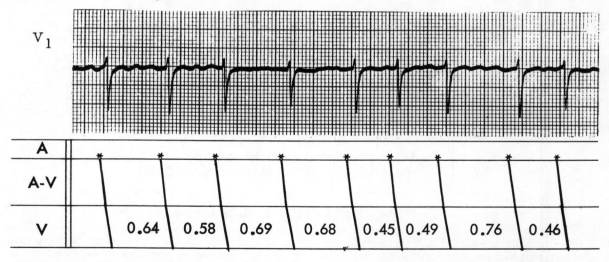

Fig. 107. Atrial fibrillation. There is a grossly irregular ventricular response, with R-R intervals varying from .76 to .45 second. The base line shows fibrillatory wave activity with some variation in the depth of the waves.

242

lation is usually 140 to 200 beats per minute, but may sometimes be extremely rapid (up to but rarely exceeding 250 beats per minute), especially at its onset. With the less rapid ventricular rates, the atrial fibrillatory waves and the gross irregularity of rhythm are easily recognizable on the electrocardiogram. With digitalis therapy administered to decrease the ventricular response toward a normal heart rate, the electrocardiographic characteristics of atrial fi-

brillation become even more obvious (fig. 107). As mentioned earlier, digitalis intoxication or disease of the A-V node may make the ventricular rhythm regular because of complete heart block with a nodal or ventricular pacemaker. In these instances, the representation of atrial activity on the electrocardiogram does not change.

Carotid sinus pressure may be helpful in the diagnosis of a very rapid tachycardia due to

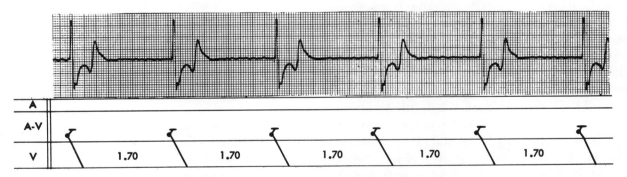

Fig. 108. Atrial fibrillation with complete heart block. The base line demonstrates fine atrial fibrillation. However, instead of the expected gross irregularity and normal or rapid heart rate, the ventricular response is slow (36 per minute) and perfectly regular. The precise pacemaker location is difficult to determine in this case, but it is probably low nodal, rather than ventricular. Atrial fibrillation with a slow and regular ventricular response indicates the presence of a high degree of heart block, which may be either pathologic or drug-induced.

243

atrial fibrillation. As in the case of atrial flutter, carotid sinus pressure may cause a transient decrease in the ventricular response, allowing the otherwise obscured atrial fibrillatory waves to be seen between the QRS complexes.

In summary, the differential diagnosis of rapid atrial arrhythmias includes sinus tachycardia, paroxysmal atrial tachycardia, atrial flutter, and atrial fibrillation. While the rate of the tachycardia may occasionally be useful (at least in a statistical sense), its primary value is a negative one. For example, if discrete atrial activity is seen at a relatively slower tachycardia (120 to 140), atrial fibrillation is excluded and atrial flutter may also be excluded. Constant electrocardiographic monitoring during carotid sinus pressure is an extremely helpful technique. Sinus tachycardia will slow and then gradually speed up again after carotid sinus pressure. Paroxysmal atrial tachycardia is either uninfluenced by carotid sinus pressure or will abruptly revert to a normal sinus rhythm; and atrial flutter and fibrillation exhibit a decrease in ventricular response, often rendering flutter or fibrillatory waves obvious during the slower rate.

This is a temporary response; the rate rapidly returns to its prior level.

Atrial Premature Beats. These are common and occur both with and without identifiable heart disease. Frequent (often multifocal) premature atrial contractions often precede the onset of atrial tachycardia or atrial flutter or fibrillation. On the other hand, occasional unifocal atrial premature systoles are often seen in the absence of heart disease, sometimes being precipitated by excesses of caffeine, tobacco, or alcohol or by fatigue.

Electrocardiographically, the premature atrial contraction is recognized as an early P wave, frequently different in configuration from the normal P wave (fig. 109). Conduction of the premature impulse, with a resulting QRS complex, may or may not occur.

The premature P-QRS is followed by a pause. There are two types of pause that occur after premature beats—the *compensatory pause* and the *noncompensatory pause*. If the time duration between the P-QRS preceding the premature beat and the P-QRS following the premature beat is equal to two normal cycles, the pause is fully *compensatory*. This occurs when the premature impulse does not interfere with the sinus node cycle. When the time duration between the P-QRS preceding and the P-QRS following the premature beat is less than two normal sinus cycles, the pause is *noncompensa-*

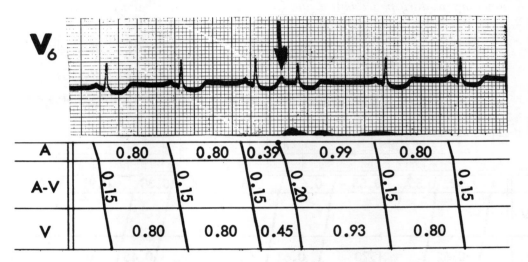

V₆					
A	0.80	0.80	0.39	0.99	0.80
A-V	0.15	0.15	0.15 / 0.20	0.15	0.15
V	0.80	0.80	0.45	0.93	0.80

FIG. 109. Premature atrial contraction. The fourth QRS is early and of the same configuration as the other complexes. The differential diagnosis lies between premature atrial beat and premature A-V nodal beat. There is an abrupt upward deflection at the end of the T wave of the complex preceding the premature beat. This deflection is not present in the T waves of the other complexes on the tracing and is the representation of the superimposed P wave of the premature atrial beat. The pause following the premature beat is noncompensatory (less than two full cycle lengths from the P wave before the early P wave to the P wave after it—see text), which is characteristic of premature atrial beats. The P-R interval of the premature complex is prolonged because of residual refractoriness in parts of the A-V conduction system at the time of the early beat.

245

tory. This occurs when the premature impulse travels retrogradely to the sinus node and discharges it early, thus interrupting the sinus cycle. *A noncompensatory pause is the rule* following a premature atrial beat, although compensatory pauses do occur rarely (fig. 110).

When a premature impulse is conducted the resulting ventricular complex either may be per-

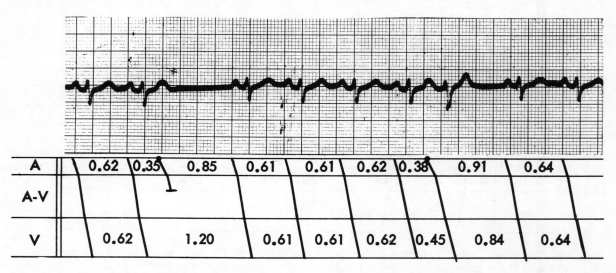

A	0.62	0.35	0.85	0.61	0.61	0.62	0.38	0.91	0.64
A-V									
V	0.62		1.20	0.61	0.61	0.62	0.45	0.84	0.64

FIG. 110. Premature atrial beats, conducted and non-conducted. The T waves of the second and sixth QRS complexes on the tracing are slightly deformed by the P waves of two premature atrial contractions. The first premature atrial impulse is not conducted to the ventricles; thus, there is no QRS complex following it. The second premature atrial impulse is conducted, and a QRS complex with slight aberration of conduction (Chapter 15) follows the early P wave. It is noteworthy that both premature atrial beats are followed by fully compensatory pauses, rather than the noncompensatory pause which usually follows premature atrial beats.

fectly normal in configuration or may be aberrantly conducted, with an abnormal configuration. (See Chapter 15 for discussion of aberrant ventricular conduction.) When the premature atrial contraction occurs close enough to the preceding beat or when there is some degree of A-V block present, the atrial impulse may not be conducted to the ventricles (fig. 110). Thus, an early abnormal P wave, not followed by a QRS, is seen on the electrocardiogram, and a pause follows which is usually noncompensatory. A premature atrial contraction may occur during the inscription of the T waves of the preceding beat, and the abnormal P wave may be difficult or impossible to recognize; and the differentiation of the premature atrial beat from a nodal premature beat or from a ventricular premature beat (if aberrant ventricular conduction has occurred) may be difficult. Frequently, however, the P wave obscured by the T wave sufficiently deforms the T wave to make its presence identifiable (fig. 109). For this reason, when premature atrial beats are suspected, but P waves cannot be identified, careful study of the T wave contour of the preceding and subsequent beats may reveal the diagnosis.

When an inverted early P wave is present in Lead II and is followed by a normal QRS with a P-R interval of .12 second or longer, differentiation between a lower atrial premature contraction and a nodal premature contraction with anterograde delay of conduction (see Chapter 14) may be impossible.

CHAPTER FOURTEEN

A-V Junctional Rhythm Disturbances

A-V Junctional Pacemaker Function. The A-V junction is equipped with its own pacemaker function, at an intrinsic rate of 40 to 60 beats per minute. Teleologically, this provides a safety mechanism that will take over the pacing function of the heart should the higher (S-A nodal or atrial) centers fail. Conversely, since the normal A-V junctional rate is slower than the normal sinus rate, the junctional pacemaker function will not disturb the physiological pattern of impulse formation and conduction under normal circumstances. In the presence of pathological or pharmacological abnormalities, however, there may be inappropriate usurping of pacemaker function by this mechanism.

Junctional Escape Beats. When the normal sinus mechanism slows sufficiently or fails completely, the A-V junction will escape and pace the heart—unless, of course, the A-V junction is diseased or suppressed to the extent that it cannot function in this capacity. Activation of this escape mechanism may occur in the absence of disease, as in the well-trained athlete whose physiologic bradycardia may become slow enough that nodal escape beats occur. Excessive vagal tone due to pharmacologic effects may also induce junctional escape. Among diseases associated with junctional escape mechanisms are sinus bradycardia in the course of acute inferior myocardial infarction and any degenerative or inflammatory lesion which may interfere with sinus node or atrial pacemaker function.

The electrocardiographic representation of A-V junctional escape is easily recognized (fig. 111). Since the pathway of conduction of the impulse through the ventricles is usually normal,

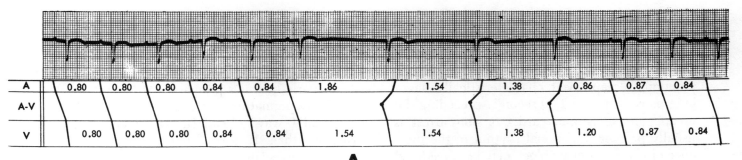

A	0.80	0.80	0.80	0.84	0.84	1.86		1.54	1.38	0.86	0.87	0.84
A-V												
V	0.80	0.80	0.80	0.84	0.84	1.54	1.54	1.38	1.20	0.87	0.84	

A

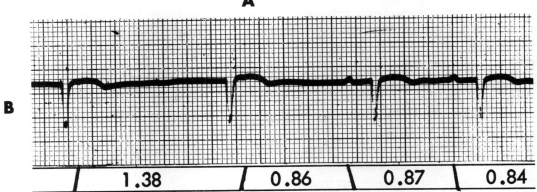

1.38	0.86	0.87	0.84

B

FIG. 111. Sinus pause or arrest with junctional escape. (A) The first six complexes show normal sinus rhythm. A long pause (1.54 seconds) follows the sixth complex, and the pause is terminated by an *escape beat.* The junction escapes twice more before a normal sinus mechanism returns. The escape beats have the same QRS configuration as the sinus beats. (B) The top of the T wave of each junctional beat is slightly deformed by a very small negative deflection not present on the T waves of the normally conducted sinus beats. This negative deflection is an inverted P wave conducted retrograde from the junctional pacemaker.

249

the QRS complexes of junctional escape beats are usually identical (or nearly so) to the normally conducted sinus beats on the tracing. In addition to a normal QRS configuration, the junctional escape beat characteristically has a long pause (at least 1.00 second) preceding the escape; and sinus bradycardia, or sinus arrest, is usually present. Junctional rhythm in the presence of complete heart block may be considered an escape mechanism. However, junctional rhythm is unusual with complete heart block because the disease of the A-V junction causing heart block is often extensive enough to destroy pacemaker function or to block conduction of a junctional impulse.

Premature Junctional Beats. Inflammatory, ischemic, pharmacologic, or "idiopathic" lesions of the A-V node or His bundle may be associated with premature junctional beats. The complexes often have an identical configuration as those of the normal sinus beats. However, instead of following a pause or occurring in association with sinus bradycardia or sinus arrest, junctional extrasystoles may occur at any heart rate and occur early (i.e., a short interval preceding the junctional beat).

Careful search for P waves should be made if junctional premature beats are suspected. When a normal anterograde P wave (with a normal or long P-R interval) is seen to precede an early beat, the early beat is a premature atrial systole rather than a premature junctional systole. When an inverted P wave (Lead II, III, or aV$_F$) occurring less than .12 second before the premature QRS is associated with the premature beat of normal configuration, it is usually positive evidence of junctional premature systole (figs. 112 and 113). The inverted P wave may precede or follow the QRS complex, or it may be buried in the QRS complex and be unidentifiable on the standard electrocardiogram. In general, an inverted P wave preceding the QRS indicates an extrasystolic focus high in the A-V junction, an inverted P wave following the QRS indicates an extrasystolic focus low in the junction, and a P wave concealed in the QRS indicates mid-junctional focus (fig. 114). Conversely, if the inverted P wave precedes the QRS complex by .12 second or more, it may be a premature atrial beat from a focus low in the atrium.

It may be difficult or impossible to differenti-

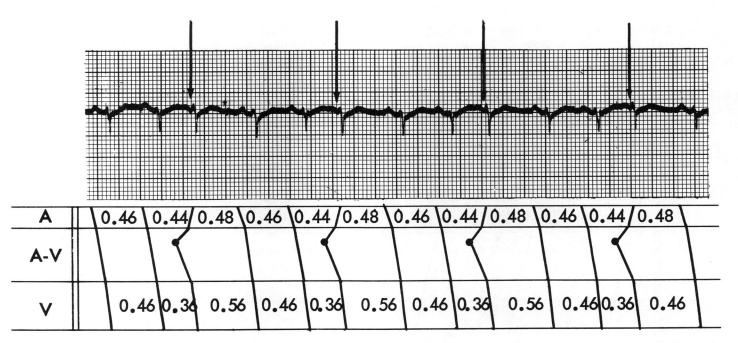

A	0.46	0.44	0.48	0.46	0.44	0.48	0.46	0.44	0.48	0.46	0.44	0.48
A-V												
V	0.46	0.36	0.56	0.46	0.36	0.56	0.46	0.36	0.56	0.46	0.36	0.46

Fig. 112. Junctional premature beats with fixed coupling intervals. Every third beat is a premature beat (the third, sixth, ninth, and twelfth complexes). These beats occur *early* and have the same configuration as the QRS complexes of the sinus beats. In addition, the premature beats are *preceded by inverted P waves* (arrows) beginning *.04 second before the QRS*. Since the P-R interval is less than .12 second, it may be concluded that the P waves are conducted retrograde from the focus of the junctional pacemaker. Since the P wave precedes the QRS, the site of the pacemaker is probably high in the A-V junction. The P-R intervals of the sinus beats are constant at .14 second, and the premature junctional beats are followed by a fully compensatory pause.

251

ate a premature junctional beat conducted with ventricular aberration from a ventricular pre- mature beat. However, an inverted P wave in a lead normally having upright P waves (Lead II

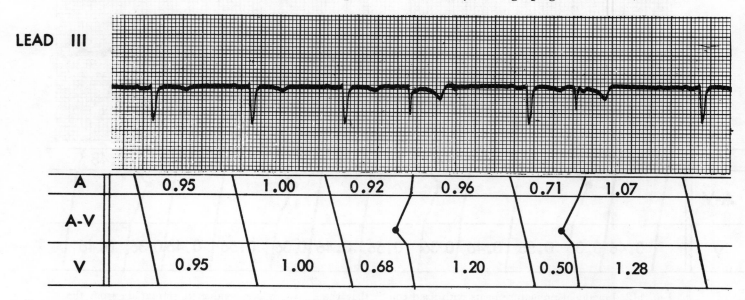

LEAD III

A	0.95	1.00	0.92	0.96	0.71	1.07
A-V						
V	0.95	1.00	0.68	1.20	0.50	1.28

Fig. 113. Junctional extrasystoles. The fourth and sixth beats occur early and are similar to the normally conducted beats. The sixth beat is followed by an inverted P wave buried in the ST segment, and the fourth beat is deformed at the ST junction by another inverted P wave. The A-V diagram demonstrates that the junctional extrasystoles have both anterograde and retro- grade conduction, with the retrograde conduction being responsible for the inverted P waves. The variable cou- pling interval between the normal beats and the extra- systoles (.68 and .50 second) suggests that junctional parasystole possibly may be producing this extrasystolic activity (see Chapter 18).

or aV_F) preceding a QRS complex of abnormal configuration with a P-R interval of less than .12 second makes the diagnosis of junctional premature beat with aberration probable. The atria would not be discharged before the ventricles by an impulse originating in the ventricles.

Junctional Tachycardia. If a junctional pacemaker usurps the pacing function of the heart at a rate in excess of 100 per minute, junctional tachycardia is present. However, if the rate is between 60 and 100 beats per minute, tachycardia is not present by definition, but as the normal intrinsic rate of the junctional pacemaker is below 60 beats per minute, a junctional rate between 60 and 100 per minute is abnormally rapid for this pacemaker. Thus, this rhythm should be considered as an *accelerated junctional rhythm*, which implies an abnormality but not a *tachycardia*.

The electrocardiographic criteria for junctional tachycardia are the same as those for premature nodal beats insofar as QRS morphology and P-R relationships are concerned (fig. 115). The heart rate must exceed 100 beats per minute. Persistent junctional tachycardia presents no problem of definition. Intermittent groups of junctional premature beats do pose a problem in terminology, however, and different authorities accept several different numbers of consecutive beats as constituting a burst of nodal tachycardia. Whether three, four, five or more consecutive junctional beats constitute the minimum for diagnosis of a "burst of junctional tachycardia" is not critical, as long as the significance of their presence is understood.

A-V Dissociation. Much of the confusion regarding A-V dissociation is due to conflicting terms and definitions. Our definition is chosen for its simplicity, but different terms and definitions are presented by others (see discussion of topic by Marriott).

A-V dissociation usually occurs by one, or by a combination, of two mechanisms—either by an abnormal slowing of the sinus node to a rate below the intrinsic A-V junctional rate or by an increase of the intrinsic A-V junctional rate above the sinus node pacemaker rate. In both instances, the common denominator is a junctional rate faster than the sinus rate (fig. 116). Two different pacemakers thus drive the heart—

253

Fig. 114. Relationships between P waves and QRS complexes in junctional rhythm, as related to site of impulse formation and presence of impaired conduction.

(A) With an A-V nodal focus high in the junction and normal forward and backward conduction, a retrograde P wave precedes the QRS complex, and the interval between the P wave onset and the QRS onset is less than .12 second. With a midjunctional focus and normal conduction, the retrograde P wave is buried in the QRS complex. With a low junctional focus and normal conduction, a retrograde P wave follows the QRS complex.

(B) If anterograde (forward) conduction delay or partial block (labeled AB) or retrograde (backward) conduction delay or partial block (labeled RB) are present, the normal time relationships may be changed or exaggerated. For instance, a high junctional focus with *anterograde block* may produce an interval between the P wave and QRS in excess of .12 second. This makes differentiation of A-V nodal from coronary sinus rhythm (low atrial) impossible. When a high nodal focus is accompanied by *retrograde block*, on the other hand, the resulting relationships of P and QRS may be the same as seen with uncomplicated low junctional focus. Midjunctional focus with anterograde block looks like high junctional focus and with retrograde block looks like low junctional focus. Finally, low junctional foci with anterograde block may look like high or midjunctional and with retrograde block, exaggerate the usual low junctional relationship. *It must be emphasized that these situations with partial block are extremely difficult to diagnose. Thus, the terms high, mid-, and low junctional beats are usually used without consideration of the presence of block; and, for practical purposes, they are merely a convenient method to express and/or explain the P wave and QRS complex relationships in a junctional beat. They have little value in truly localizing the site of impulse formation.*

254

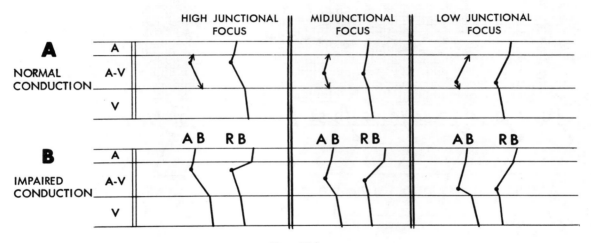

HIGH JUNCTIONAL
FOCUS

MIDJUNCTIONAL
FOCUS

LOW JUNCTIONAL
FOCUS

A

NORMAL
CONDUCTION

A

A-V

V

B

IMPAIRED
CONDUCTION

A

A-V

V

A B   R B   A B   R B   A B   R B

F_{IG}. 114

a sinus pacemaker controls the atria and an A-V junctional pacemaker controls the ventricles. While the junctional pacemaker is the faster, the rates of the two pacemakers are usually fairly

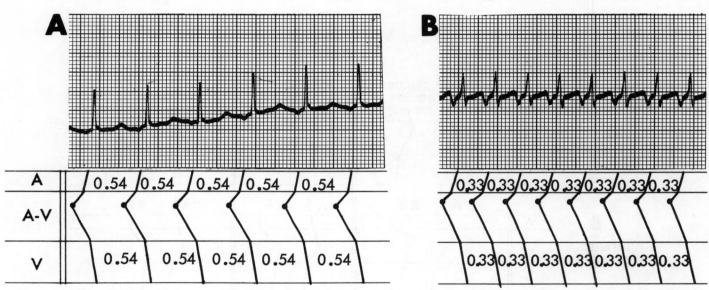

Fig. 115. Junctional tachycardia. (A) A relatively slow junctional tachycardia is demonstrated, the rate being approximately 111 beats per minute and the rhythm perfectly regular. Since the lead is standard Lead II and each QRS complex is preceded by an inverted P wave with a P-R interval of .09, the assumption may be made that retrograde activation of the atria from the junctional pacemaker is occurring. (B) A rapid junctional tachycardia is shown. The rhythm is again perfectly regular and the rate is about 182 per minute. This is also Lead II and the QRS complexes are preceded by inverted P waves with a P-R interval of .10 second, indicating retrograde atrial activation from the junctional pacemaker.

close. Were this not true, the junctional pacemaker would drive both the ventricles *and* atria and a junctional rhythm with retrograde atrial activation (as in fig. 114) would be present. However, when the rates are close together, the sinus impulses conducted into the A-V tissue interfere with retrograde conduction of the junctional impulses, and thus the two pacemakers continue to function (fig. 116). When concomitant partial A-V block is also present, however, the rates of the two pacemakers may be more divergent.

The rhythm in A-V dissociation is basically regular, but the regularity is interrupted by *capture beats*. Remembering that A-V dissociation is not, in itself, a form of *heart block* and that A-V conduction is therefore usually potentially normal, a P wave occurring at a time when the

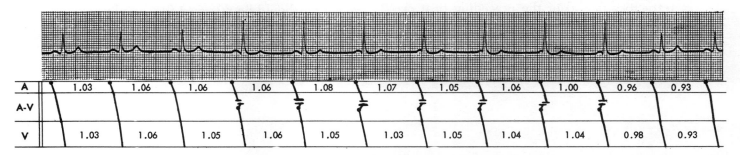

A	1.03	1.06	1.06	1.06	1.08	1.07	1.05	1.06	1.00	0.96	0.93
A-V											
V	1.03	1.06	1.05	1.06	1.05	1.03	1.05	1.04	1.04	0.98	0.93

Fig. 116. A-V dissociation due to sinus bradycardia and junctional escape. The first three complexes are normal sinus beats with normal A-V conduction. The heart rate is just below 60 beats per minute. The fourth beat is a junctional escape beat with a slightly different QRS morphology and shorter interval between the onset of the P wave and the onset of the QRS complex than the preceding sinus beats. The sinus node rate slows a little more during the next few cycles and the junctional escape rate remains relatively constant, perpetuating the A-V dissociation. As the sinus rate then increases, the P waves emerge from the QRS complexes and finally *recapture* the ventricles (last two complexes). The atrial (higher) pacemaker is slower than the junctional (lower) pacemaker during the period of dissociation, permitting the A-V dissociation to occur.

257

conducting tissue is no longer refractory from the preceding junctional impulse, and before the next junctional impulse occurs, may be conducted and depolarize the ventricles. This is called a *capture beat* and is recognized as an early beat, preceded by a P wave, which occurs beyond the refractory period of the preceding QRS complex. The P-R interval of a capture beat is normal unless (1) the P wave occurs in the relative refractory period of the preceding beat or (2) first-degree heart block coexists with the A-V dissociation.

It should be clearly understood that, while the atria and ventricles are hemodynamically and pathologically "dissociated" in complete heart block, the term "A-V dissociation," as we are using it, refers to a physiologic dissociation due to a lower pacemaker having a higher rate than a higher pacemaker. Heart block may or may not coexist with "A-V dissociation," but heart block is not an essential feature of it. To avoid confusion, we feel that the term A-V dissociation should be reserved for the physiologic dissociation described and should not be used in reference to the dissociation of complete heart block.

CHAPTER FIFTEEN
Ventricular Arrhythmias

Ventricular Pacemaker Function. If all the higher pacemakers fail to function, the intrinsic pacemaker activity of the ventricles will pace the heart at a spontaneous discharge rate of 20 to 40 beats per minute. Again, therefore, a lower pacemaker is present with a slower intrinsic rate than the higher level pacemakers, and the slower rate prevents the lower pacemaker from usurping pacemaker function under normal conditions.

Ventricular Escape Beats. Ventricular escape beating occurs most commonly in complete heart block (see Chapter 17). In this situation, even though the higher and faster atrial pacemaker may be intact and functioning, none of the impulses reach the ventricles because of the A-V block. Thus, the dominant rhythm becomes a ventricular escape rhythm or idioventricular rhythm. Ventricular escape beats also occasionally occur during carotid sinus pressure for reversion of paroxysmal atrial tachycardia. Other than these two situations, ventricular escape beats are uncommon, as the faster A-V nodal pacemaker tends to escape during a sinus pause.

Premature Ventricular Beats. Premature ventricular beats are extremely common in all age groups, both with and without demonstrable organic heart disease. The patient may be completely asymptomatic or may experience only annoying symptoms such as palpitations. Or the premature beats may be a cause for serious concern to both patient and physician—depending upon the setting in which they occur and upon their frequency.

Electrocardiographically, the characteristics of premature ventricular contractions are (1)

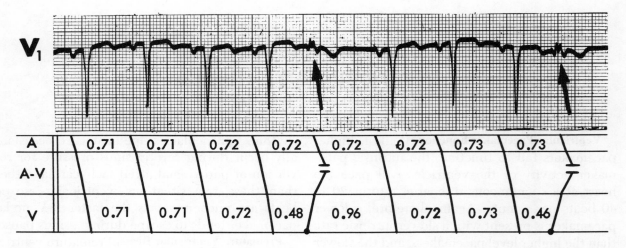

V₁								
A	0.71	0.71	0.72	0.72	0.72	0.72	0.73	0.73
A-V								
V	0.71	0.71	0.72	0.48	0.96	0.72	0.73	0.46

FIG. 117. Premature ventricular contractions. There is a normal sinus rhythm, with the fifth and ninth beats (arrows) occurring early and having a markedly different configuration from that of the normal sinus beats. They have a QRS duration in excess of .12 second and are not preceded by discernible P waves. Both premature beats are followed by a fully compensatory pause; that is, the two sinus cycles from the second to the fourth beat measure 1.43 seconds and the two cycles from the fourth to the sixth beat (which includes the abnormal fifth beat) measure 1.44 seconds. All these characteristics favor the diagnosis of premature ventricular beats. Finally, it can be positively demonstrated that the sinus node cycle is not interrupted. The P-P interval of the cycle preceding the first premature beat measures .72 second in duration. If one measures .72 second from the P wave of the fourth beat, it is seen to coincide with the inverted wave at the beginning of the ST segment of the premature beat, which exactly matches the configuration of the normal P waves in this lead. Thus, the P wave originates in the sinus node and discharges the atria but is not conducted to the ventricles. The A-V diagram indicates the interference at the A-V level. Finally, measuring from the P wave at the end of the premature beat to the next P wave demonstrates the expected .72 second length of the cycle.

early beats which (2) have a QRS duration greater than .12 second and bizarre contour and (3) are followed by a fully compensatory pause (fig. 117). The fully compensatory pause is due to the fact that the sinus node rhythm is not interrupted by retrograde conduction from the premature beat. Thus, two full sinus cycles enclose the premature ventricular contraction.

Another type of premature ventricular contraction (fig. 118) is the *interpolated* beat. The interpolated premature ventricular contraction occurs between two consecutive normal sinus beats and does not interrupt the basic sinus rhythm. Thus, there is no pause and this is truly an "extra" systole. The interpolated premature ventricular beat usually occurs in the setting of a relatively slow sinus rate, because with a rapid sinus rate, the ventricles and/or conducting system would be refractory to the first sinus impulse following the premature beat (fig. 118).

A simple premature ventricular beat is usually related to the preceding sinus beat by *fixed coupling;* that is, each premature beat on a given electrocardiogram occurs at a constant time interval from the onset of the sinus beat immediately preceding it. On the other hand, when the coupling interval is variable, a parasystole may be the mechanism of the premature contractions (see Chapter 18).

Differentiation of Premature Ventricular Beats from Premature Supraventricular Beats with Aberrant Ventricular Conduction. A premature atrial or premature A-V nodal beat occurring soon enough after the preceding sinus beat may reach the ventricular conducting tissue before it has fully recovered from the preceding beat. Since recovery is not perfectly uniform, some areas of the ventricular conducting system may be partially refractory, while other areas of the system may be able to conduct normally. The activation impulse may thus take an aberrant pathway through the ventricles, rather than follow the normal pathway and sequence of depolarization. Electrocardiographically, this presents as a bizarre, widened QRS complex (fig. 119), often of a right bundle branch block type of configuration. The aberration is an inversely variable function of the time since the last depolarization, and so there may be anything from a minimal change in QRS duration to a com-

261

pletely bizarre beat which mimics premature ventricular activity. Differentiation of premature atrial or nodal beats with marked aberration from premature ventricular beats may be difficult or sometimes impossible. If a premature atrial beat is seen preceding the early, bizarre QRS, aberration is the cause. However, premature atrial beats are often difficult to iden-

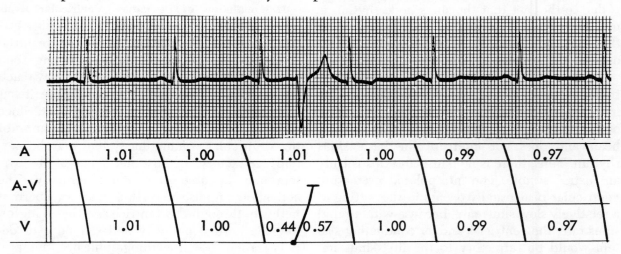

A	1.01	1.00	1.01	1.00	0.99	0.97
A-V						
V	1.01	1.00	0.44 / 0.57	1.00	0.99	0.97

FIG. 118. Interpolated premature ventricular contraction. The P waves and QRS complexes on the tracing are quite constant at a rate of about 60 beats per minute. There is a wide, abnormally configured premature QRS between the third and fourth sinus beats, and the premature beat does not interrupt the sinus rhythm. The P wave of the fourth beat (the one following the premature beat) is difficult to identify in the descending limb of the T wave of the premature beat, but its presence can be inferred from the fact that the beat following the premature beat is normal in configuration and does not break the sinus cycle sequence (as indicated in the A-V diagram). Finally, note the phenomenon of postextrasystolic T wave inversion in the first normal beat after the premature beat.

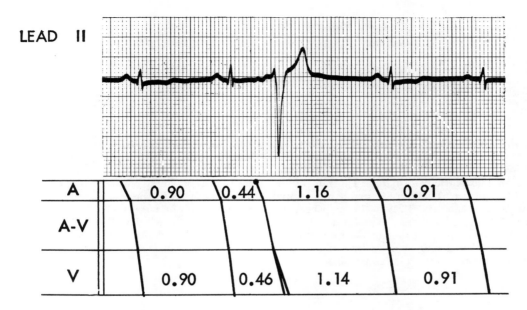

LEAD II

A	0.90	0.44	1.16	0.91
A-V				
V	0.90	0.46	1.14	0.91

FIG. 119. Premature atrial impulse with aberrant ventricular conduction. The first two complexes on the tracing are normal sinus beats. The P waves, QRS complexes, and P-R intervals are normal, and the rate is 67 per minute. The T wave of the second complex is deformed by an abnormal, biphasic, early P wave which is followed by a QRS complex of distinctly abnormal configuration. Because of the presence of the premature P wave coupled to the abnormal QRS complex by a normal P-R interval, the diagnosis of premature atrial impulse with aberration of ventricular conduction may be made. This occurs because of refractoriness in parts of the A-V junction at the time when the premature impulse arrives, causing an abnormal pathway of conduction. In the case of a premature A-V *junctional* beat with aberrant conduction, the differentiation from premature ventricular beat may be more difficult or impossible— depending on the P wave relationship.

263

Fig. 120. Ventricular tachycardia. (A) Complete heart block is present, as manifested by the absence of any relationship between the P waves and QRS complexes and an idioventricular rhythm. The rate of the idioventricular rhythm, however, is much more rapid than the normal escape rate of a ventricular pacemaker (P-R interval of basic rhythm = .86 second, rate = 70 per minute). Therefore, even though the rate does not conform to the usual definition of tachycardia (rate = 100), it is an abnormal rate for this pacemaker and is therefore called an *accelerated ventricular rhythm*. Note, too, the irregular extrasystolic activity present. (B) Ventricular tachycardia with a rate of 136 per minute is present. Complete heart block is still present and a number of the P waves are easily seen. Since the P-P intervals are quite constant, the presence of the other P waves is inferred. The P waves and QRS complexes are completely independent of each other because of the complete heart block.

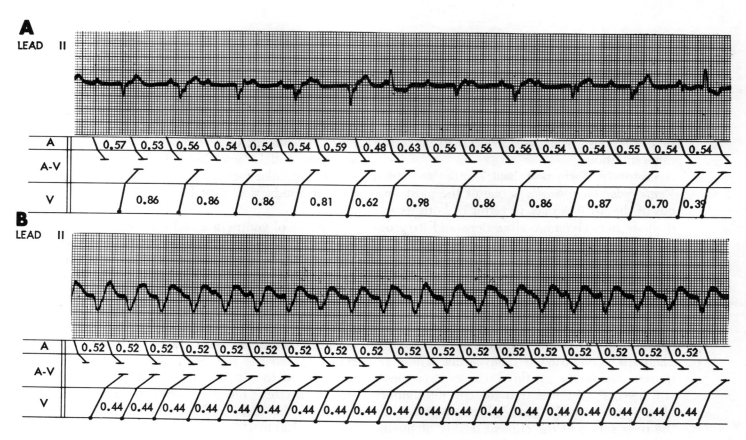

A

LEAD II

| A | 0.57 | 0.53 | 0.56 | 0.54 | 0.54 | 0.54 | 0.59 | 0.48 | 0.63 | 0.56 | 0.56 | 0.56 | 0.54 | 0.54 | 0.55 | 0.54 | 0.54 |

A-V

| V | 0.86 | 0.86 | 0.86 | 0.81 | 0.62 | 0.98 | 0.86 | 0.86 | 0.87 | 0.70 | 0.39 |

B

LEAD II

| A | 0.52 | 0.52 | 0.52 | 0.52 | 0.52 | 0.52 | 0.52 | 0.52 | 0.52 | 0.52 | 0.52 | 0.52 | 0.52 | 0.52 | 0.52 | 0.52 | 0.52 |

A-V

| V | 0.44 | 0.44 | 0.44 | 0.44 | 0.44 | 0.44 | 0.44 | 0.44 | 0.44 | 0.44 | 0.44 | 0.44 | 0.44 | 0.44 | 0.44 | 0.44 | 0.44 | 0.44 |

FIG. 120

tify because they may be small and fall in the T waves of preceding complexes. In addition, aberrant conduction often occurs in the presence of atrial fibrillation. Therefore, it is frequently necessary to rely upon other criteria, based for the most part on QRS morphology and certain time relationships (see Marriott), to make the differentiation.

Ventricular Tachycardia and Ventricular Flutter. *Ventricular tachycardia* is one of the most serious of the arrhythmias, in terms of both its immediate hemodynamic alterations and its prognostic significance. It occurs most frequently with coronary artery occlusion or as a manifestation of digitalis intoxication and/or electrolyte disturbances. Sustained ventricular tachycardia generally requires prompt therapy.

Various authorities require different numbers of consecutive ectopic ventricular beats for the diagnosis of ventricular tachycardia. These requirements begin at three consecutive beats and increase. We feel that the specific number of ectopic ventricular beats is less important than the recognition of the clinical setting of the arrhythmia and an understanding of its prognos-

tic implications. The electrocardiographic representation of a burst of ventricular tachycardia (see fig. 120) is a cluster of wide (greater than .12 second), bizarre QRS complexes interrupting the basic cardiac rhythm. A paroxysm of sustained ventricular tachycardia may sometimes be difficult to recognize. The complexes are wide and bizarre, but differentiation from supraventricular tachycardia with aberrant ventricular conduction may be difficult or impossible.

The rate of ventricular tachycardia may be as fast as 180 to 200, but may also be much slower. The same problem of definition exists with ventricular rhythms as with nodal rhythms when the heart rate is less than 100, but greater than the intrinsic rate of the ventricular pacemaker (i.e., greater than 40 per minute). It is best to reserve the term "tachycardia" for instances when the rate is greater than 100 per minute and to use the term "accelerated ventricular rhythm" for rates between 40 and 100. Ventricular tachycardia commonly occurs at a rate of 130 to 180 per minute, which places it in the same range of rates as most supraventricular tachycardias. The rhythm of ventricular tachycardia may be somewhat irregular, but the degree of irregularity is often minimal, similar to the slight irregularity occasionally seen in some of the supraventricular tachycardias. P waves may be of help in the differential diagnosis if they can be identified (fig. 120).

Ventricular flutter probably is not a distinct entity, but an extreme end of the spectrum of ventricular tachycardia, bridging it with ventricular fibrillation. Ventricular flutter is characterized by very regular and smooth ventricular wave forms at a rate of 150 to 300 per minute (fig. 121). P waves are not evident.

Ventricular Fibrillation. Ventricular fibrillation is incompatible with life, since it is an uncoordinated depolarization of the ventricular musculature which does not result in an effective cardiac output. Now that effective electrical defibrillation devices are available, it is often a treatable arrhythmia if cardiac output is maintained by external cardiac massage until defibrillation can be performed.

The electrocardiogram shows irregular wave-

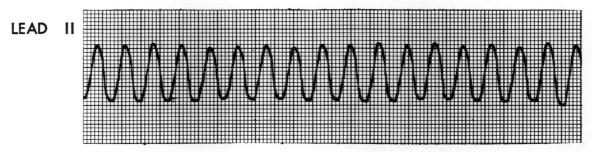

LEAD II

FIG. 121. Ventricular flutter. This rhythm forms a clinical bridge between ventricular tachycardia and ventricular fibrillation. There are very smooth, regular wave forms at a rate of 207 per minute. The patient still had a cardiac output at the time of this event, but it was markedly reduced. This rhythm rarely lasts more than a few seconds to a minute, tending to progress rapidly to ventricular fibrillation or to revert to ventricular tachycardia or other rhythm.

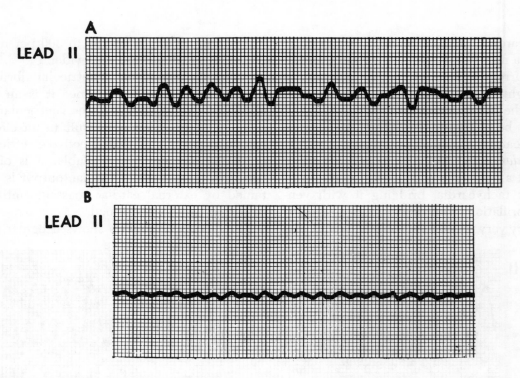

FIG. 122. Ventricular fibrillation. This rhythm is incompatible with life since it represents uncoordinated ventricular activity with no cardiac output. It is, however, frequently treatable, the success of treatment depending on the setting in which it occurs. (A) *Coarse ventricular fibrillation*. Note the irregular wave-form activity. (B) *Fine ventricular fibrillation*. This type of pattern frequently precedes the complete cessation of electrical activity at the time of biological death of the heart and is very difficult to defibrillate.

form activity (fig. 122). The waves may range from quite coarse to very fine, the latter approaching a straight line. More coarse waves tend to be seen at the onset, with fine waves preceding the cessation of all electrical activity at the time of biological death of the cardiac muscle cells.

Ventricular fibrillation should be differentiated from *cardiac standstill,* in which no identifiable ventricular activity is seen. In cardiac standstill the electrocardiogram is simply a straight line or occasionally a straight line with P waves. Ventricular fibrillation probably accounts for most sudden deaths in the course of acute myocardial infarction, whereas cardiac standstill is probably more common in long-standing degenerative or ischemic heart disease without identifiable acute precipitating cause of death and also in acute anoxic states.

CHAPTER SIXTEEN

The Differential Diagnosis of a Tachycardia

Differentiation between Supraventricular and Ventricular Tachycardias

It is common to be confronted with the problem of the differential diagnosis of a tachycardia. Accuracy is important since the various tachycardias are treated differently and have different prognostic significance. Often the diagnosis is clear immediately upon examining the patient or briefly studying the electrocardiogram. On the other hand, however, it may occasionally be almost impossible to make a definitive conclusion about the nature of a tachycardia— even with the use of the most sophisticated techniques available. Nevertheless, with the careful application of a few general rules, most of the tachycardias can be identified.

When the supraventricular tachycardias (sinus tachycardia, paroxysmal atrial tachycardia, atrial flutter with 2:1 ventricular response, atrial fibrillation with rapid ventricular response, and A-V nodal tachycardia) have normal conduction through the ventricles, distinction between them (as a group) and ventricular tachycardia is usually simple, since the QRS morphology will be normal. In ventricular tachycardia, however, the QRS complex is always widened beyond .12 second and is of abnormal configuration. But when supraventricular tachycardia with coexistent bundle branch block occurs or when supraventricular tachycardia is accompanied by ventricular aberration, QRS morphology is of

270

little help in making the distinction. Thus, a normal QRS complex indicates supraventricular tachycardia, whereas a wide, abnormal QRS may be seen with either supraventricular or ventricular tachycardia.

P wave characteristics may aid in diagnosis. Upright P waves in Leads II, III, and aV$_F$ with a 1:1 relationship to QRS complexes indicate a supraventricular (sinus or atrial) tachycardia and inverted P waves in these leads (which precede the QRS) also indicate supraventricular tachycardia (low atrial or A-V nodal). Inverted P waves following a QRS complex are characteristic of both supraventricular ("low nodal") and ventricular tachycardia. Upright P waves without fixed relationship to the QRS complexes are of limited value, since dissociation between the P waves and QRS complexes may occur in both supraventricular (nodal) and ventricular tachycardias.

The rhythm is frequently of value. Ventricular tachycardia may be somewhat irregular; however, the degree of this irregularity is often small and may occur to almost the same extent with some of the supraventricular tachycardias.

Nevertheless, a tachycardia with wide, bizarre QRS complexes and some irregularity and with no fixed P-R relationship strongly favors ventricular tachycardia over supraventricular tachycardia. When no P waves are seen, with a somewhat irregular tachycardia and wide QRS complexes, atrial fibrillation with aberrant conduction or bundle branch block may be present. This is especially difficult to differentiate from ventricular tachycardia when the rate is rapid.

The range of rates of ventricular and supraventricular tachycardias overlap, making rate of limited value in the differential diagnosis. Carotid sinus pressure, which usually has no effect on the rate of ventricular tachycardia, but does affect rate in most of the supraventricular tachycardias, may aid in the differential diagnosis.

The differentiation of supraventricular tachycardia with bundle branch block or with aberrant conduction from ventricular tachycardia is very important and frequently impossible with standard electrocardiography. In this setting, some of the more sophisticated diagnostic techniques, such as an esophageal or transvenous right atrial lead, are indicated. These leads will

Fɪɢ. 123. Sinus tachycardia with carotid sinus pressure. The first 6 seconds (top tracing) of the electrocardiogram demonstrates a typical sinus tachycardia at a rate of 136 per minute. The P-P and R-R intervals are constant at .44 second, and the P-R interval is constant. When carotid sinus pressure is applied at the time of the first arrow (second strip of the tracing), the rate slows progressively. When the carotid sinus pressure is stopped at the time of the second arrow (third strip of the tracing), the rate progressively increases until it reaches the original rate of 136 per minute at the end of the fourth strip of the electrocardiogram. Note also the shortening of the P waves and P-R intervals as the rate decreases and the return to their original voltage and duration after the release of pressure. This pattern of events is the same as seen in wandering pacemaker and is seen occasionally in sinus tachycardia with carotid sinus pressure.

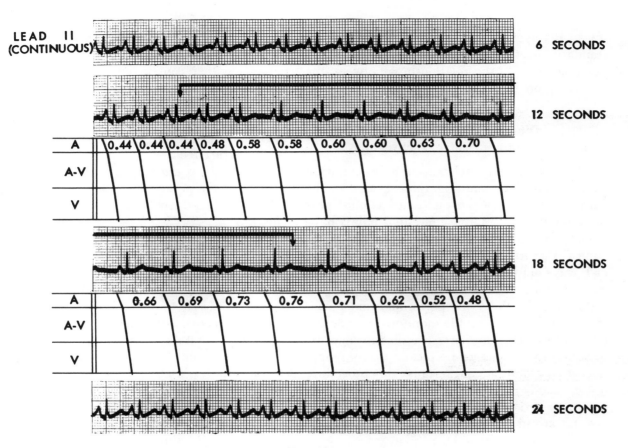

LEAD II
(CONTINUOUS)

6 SECONDS

12 SECONDS

A	0.44	0.44	0.44	0.48	0.58	0.58	0.60	0.60	0.63	0.70
A-V										
V										

18 SECONDS

A	0.66	0.69	0.73	0.76	0.71	0.62	0.52	0.48
A-V								
V								

24 SECONDS

FIG. 123

273

reveal P waves that are not identifiable on the standard electrocardiogram and thus make it possible to study the relationships between the P waves and the QRS complexes.

Differentiation of the Various Supraventricular Tachycardias

When ventricular tachycardia is ruled out on clinical and electrocardiographic evidence, the various supraventricular tachycardias must next be differentiated. Many differential points have already been listed (Chapter 13). When the clinical picture, rate, and presence and nature of P wave activity are not diagnostic, the use of carotid sinus pressure is indicated. This procedure should always be performed under constant electrocardiographic monitoring, since the effect of carotid sinus pressure on rate may be so subtle that it cannot be picked up by palpation or auscultation, and because this procedure is attended by a small but real danger of inducing more serious arrhythmias or even cardiac arrest. Carotid massage should not be performed in patients with diseased carotid arteries or with

known cerebrovascular disease and should be used only under extremely strong indications in patients with recent myocardial infarction. An alternative to the use of carotid sinus pressure is the use of the drug edrophonium (Tensilon), 10 milligrams intravenously. This will often be as effective as carotid pressure in terms of parasympathetic effect.

Sinus tachycardia responds to carotid stimulation by a temporary decrease in rate, followed by a gradual return to the prestimulation rate (fig. 123).

Paroxysmal atrial tachycardia responds in one of two ways: (1) either there is no effect at all (rarely slight slowing) or (2) there is an abrupt cessation of the tachycardia and resumption of a normal sinus rhythm (fig. 124). When paroxysmal atrial tachycardia with *varying block* (usually seen in digitalis intoxication) is present, the diagnosis is usually obvious without the use of carotid sinus pressure, since (1) the varying block permits the P waves to be seen and (2) the rhythm is irregular.

When *atrial flutter with 2:1 conduction* is present, carotid sinus pressure usually induces an increase in the degree of block, the increase being in whole-number multiples of the rate.

Thus, the conduction may become 3:1, 4:1, etc. (rate of approximately 100, 75, etc.). This in-

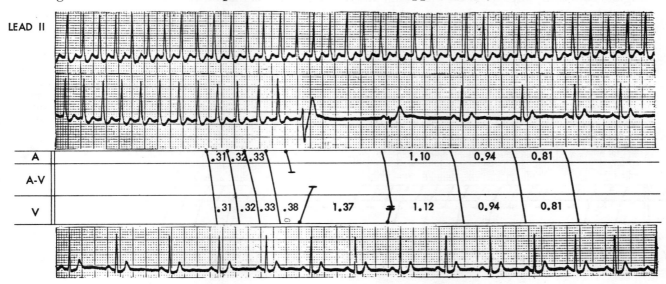

FIG. 124. Paroxysmal atrial tachycardia with carotid sinus pressure. This is a continuous tracing (Lead II) recorded during a typical attack of paroxysmal atrial tachycardia (PAT) in a nine-year-old girl without evidence of organic heart disease. In the upper strip, the rate is over 200 per minute and P waves are not identifiable. QRS duration and morphology are normal. In the middle strip of the tracing, an abrupt termination of the paroxysmal atrial tachycardia with carotid sinus pressure occurs. An extrasystole (see Chapter 15) follows the last beat of the tachycardia. This is followed by a pause terminated by a *fusion beat* (fusion between a conducted sinus beat and an escape beat—see Chapter 18). A normal sinus mechanism then resumes as seen in the rest of the second strip and in the third strip of the tracing.

crease in block is transient, and a return to the original rate fairly rapidly is the rule (fig. 125).

Atrial fibrillation similarly responds to carotid sinus pressure with an increased degree of block (fig. 126), and the slowing may make obscure fibrillatory waves demonstrable. In addition, the ventricular response will have the typical irregular response of atrial fibrillation—

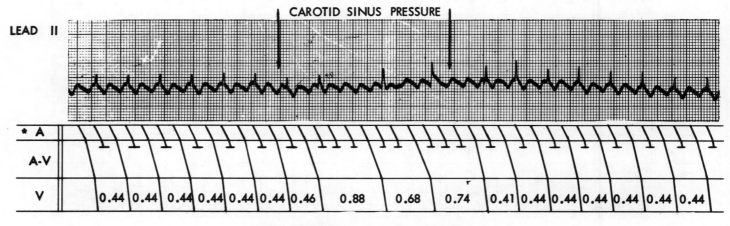

FIG. 125. Atrial flutter with 2:1 conduction and carotid sinus pressure. The effect of carotid sinus pressure in the presence of atrial flutter is demonstrated. Before carotid pressure is applied (first arrow), the interval between successive flutter waves is .22 second. The atrial rate speeds up slightly (interval about .20 second) during the application of pressure. Decrease in A-V conduction is present with consequent *temporary* slowing of the ventricular response as a result of the increased vagal tone. The decrease in conduction is frequently a whole-number multiple of the basic flutter wave intervals. During the period of slower ventricular rate, the flutter pattern becomes more obvious.

unless complete block with nodal rhythm is temporarily induced, resulting in a regular response. It is not uncommon, however, for atrial fibrillation to fail to respond to carotid sinus pressure.

Paroxysmal A-V junctional tachycardia may respond to carotid sinus pressure in the same manner as does paroxysmal atrial tachycardia—that is, by abrupt cessation of the arrhythmia. Alternatively, however, it may be unaffected by carotid sinus pressure.

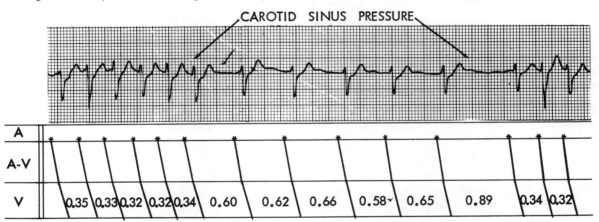

FIG. 126. Atrial fibrillation (rapid) with carotid sinus pressure. The tracing, standard Lead II, was recorded while attempting to make a diagnosis on a patient with a tachycardia. The first six QRS complexes on the electrocardiogram demonstrate a rate of about 180 per minute with slight irregularity. No P waves are visible and atrial fibrillation with rapid ventricular response was suspected. Carotid sinus massage was performed, and the rate slowed markedly to the range of 90 to 100 per minute. Irregular ventricular response and the absence of P waves is evident during the period of slower rate. Very fine atrial fibrillation waves are also seen. Very soon after the carotid sinus pressure is stopped, the rate returns to about 180 per minute.

CHAPTER SEVENTEEN

Abnormalities of Conduction and Heart Block

Disease or pharmacologic agents may affect the conduction system of the heart, causing a variable degree of conduction impairment. When the impairment becomes clinically recognizable, the condition is referred to as "block." The most easily recognized site of block clinically is in the A-V junction because the A-V junction is the electrical bridge between the P wave and the QRS complex. However, block may occur anywhere that conducting tissue is present. When it occurs in the conducting tissue distal to the bundle of His, the QRS patterns of right or left bundle branch block, or of intra-ventricular block, results (see Chapter 5).

Three degrees of block may occur—designated first, second, and third, or complete. First-degree block involves a simple prolongation of conduction time; second-degree block is inter-mittent failure of conduction; and third-degree block is complete failure of conduction. Again, it should be emphasized that these various degrees of block are most easily recognized in the A-V junction, but each may theoretically occur in a number of areas where conduction tissue is present—although not all are demonstrable by clinical electrocardiography.

First-degree A-V Block. (Fig. 127). This is a prolongation of the conduction time across the A-V junction and is manifested electrocardiographically as a constant prolongation of the P-R interval in all complexes, as measured from the onset of the P wave to the first deflection of the QRS complex. The upper limit of normal for the P-R interval varies somewhat with age and with heart rate. (See Appendix, Table 1.) The upper limit of normal in the adult patient is .20 second and is lower in children. The upper limit of normal also varies with heart rate, tending to be shorter with more rapid rates in normal persons.

Second-degree A-V Block. This occurs in two forms: the *Wenckebach* type (the more common form) and the *intermittent block* type. Both types have the characteristic of dropped beats in common, i.e., supraventricular impulses (P waves) which are not conducted through the A-V junction to discharge the ventricle.

The Wenckebach phenomenon is characterized by groups of beats ("periods") having progressively increasing P-R intervals until conduction fails completely and a beat is dropped. The dropped ventricular beat terminates each Wenckebach period (fig. 128). The greatest P-R interval *increment* (i.e., increase in P-R interval from one beat to the next) occurs between the first and second complexes of the period, and the *increment* progressively *decreases* thereafter. The R-R intervals of each cycle in the Wenckebach period progressively *decrease concomitant with the decreasing P-R interval increment* as the period continues. The pause

associated with the dropped beat is less than twice the length of the last or shortest cycle in the period. A minimum of three atrial beats with two ventricular beats are required for diagnosis of a Wenckebach phenomenon. This is called a 3:2 Wenckebach period. When four atrial beats and three ventricular beats are present, the pe-

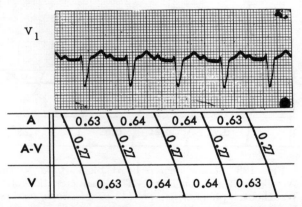

A	0.63	0.64	0.64	0.63
A-V	.27	.27	.27	.27	.27
V	0.63	0.64	0.64	0.63

FIG. 127. First-degree A-V block. The P-R interval is constant and prolonged to .27 second. When the heart rate is rapid in the presence of first-degree heart block, the P waves may be buried in the T waves of the preceding complexes. In this situation, the recognition of the pacemaker site may be difficult (see Chapter 13, fig. 103), and carotid sinus pressure may aid in diagnosis.

riod is termed 4:3 Wenckebach; and a 5:4 Wenckebach period consists of five P waves and four QRS complexes.

Intermittent type of second-degree A-V block (*Mobitz type II block*) is characterized by fixed P-R intervals with dropped beats (fig. 129). There may be a fixed and constant ratio of atrial to ventricular beats, such as every other atrial

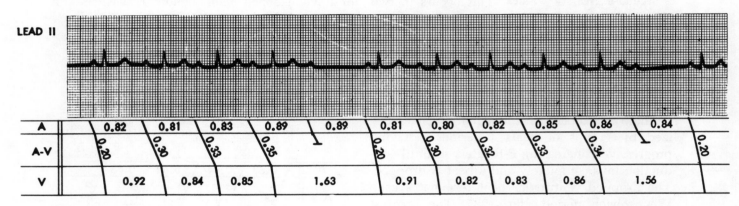

LEAD II

A	0.82	0.81	0.83	0.89	0.89	0.81	0.80	0.82	0.85	0.86	0.84	
A-V	0.20	0.30	0.33	0.35		0.20	0.30	0.32	0.33	0.34		0.20
V	0.92	0.84	0.85		1.63		0.91	0.82	0.83	0.86	1.56	

FIG. 128. Second-degree heart block, *type I* (the Wenckebach phenomenon). The characteristics of a Wenckebach phenomenon are (1) *progressively increasing* P-R intervals with (2) *progressively decreasing* R-R intervals and (3) *a pause due to a dropped beat*, the pause being less than twice the length of the last R-R interval (usually the shortest) in the period. The greatest increment of P-R interval occurs between the first and second complexes of any period, and the *increment* progressively *decreases* through the period. Thus, in the first Wenckebach period on the electrocardiogram, the first P-R interval is .20 second and the second P-R interval is .30 second, giving an increment of .30 − .20 = .10 second; the next increment is .33 − .30 = .03 second; and the last increment is .35 − .33 = .02 second. The R-R intervals decrease from .92 to .84 second. Then the last R-R interval before the pause should also decrease but does not do so in this case because of the presence of the concomitant sinus rate variation. The duration of the pause due to the dropped beat is 1.63 seconds, which is less than twice the R-R interval of the last cycle of the period (.85 × 2 = 1.70).

beat blocked(2:1 block) or three of four atrial beats blocked (4:1 block); or more commonly, the block is irregularly intermittent with blocked beats occurring variably on the tracing, without fixed pattern.

Third-degree (Complete) A-V Block. This is complete interruption of the electrical bridge between atria and ventricles. Both the atria and the ventricles have their own pacemaker, and the electrocardiogram, therefore, shows P waves and QRS complexes that are independent of each other and occurring at different rates. The ventricular rhythm is regular (fig. 130). Since most cases of complete heart block are associated with an idioventricular pacemaker, the ventricular rate is usually in the range of 30 to 40 beats per minute. Less commonly, complete heart block is present with a nodal pacemaker

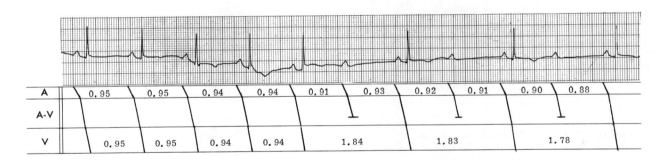

A	0.95	0.95	0.94	0.94	0.91	0.93	0.92	0.91	0.90	0.88
A-V										
V	0.95	0.95	0.94	0.94	1.84		1.83		1.78	

FIG. 129. Second-degree heart block, *type II.* The first five complexes on the tracing represent normal sinus rhythm at a rate of approximately 65 per minute. The sixth atrial beat (P wave) is abruptly blocked, and the seventh is conducted with a normal P-R interval. The patient then continues in 2:1 block to the end of the strip. Note that the P-R intervals prior to the first dropped beat are constant, as opposed to the progressive prolongation prior to the dropped beat in *type I* block (the Wenckebach phenomenon).

281

rhythm with a rate of 40 to 60 per minute. The atrial rate is usually normal or may be increased. When an electrical pacemaker is implanted, the ventricular rate is set by the physician as de-sired, often in the range of 60 to 80. The pace-maker artifact precedes each ventricular com-plex (fig. 131). The rhythm is regular.

Sinoatrial (S-A) Block. Evidence from the

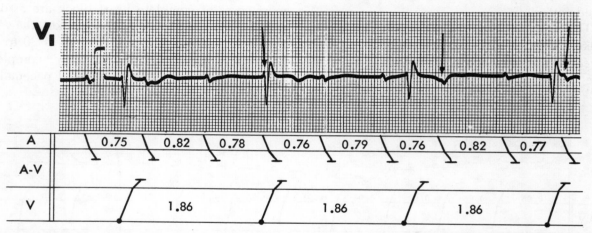

Fig. 130. Complete heart block. The ventricular rate is 32 beats per minute and the ventricular rhythm is reg-ular. There is no fixed relationship between the P waves and QRS complexes. The arrows indicate some of the P waves that fall within the QRS complexes or T waves and may be difficult to discern. There is some variation in the P-P intervals. The P wave irregularity has a defi-nite pattern; namely, the P-P interval tends to be shorter when a QRS complex falls between the two P waves and to be longer when the two P waves fall between two QRS complexes. Thus, the P-P intervals between the first and second, sixth and seventh, and eighth and ninth P waves are .75, .76, and .77 second, respectively; and the P-P intervals between the second and third, fifth and sixth, and seventh and eighth P waves are .82, .79, and .82 second, respectively. This phenomenon is called *ventriculophasic sinus arrhythmia*, a common find-ing in complete heart block with normal atrial activity.

studies of certain arrhythmias suggests that the sinus node may be separated from the atrial musculature by a "bridge" (at least functional, if not anatomic) analogous to the A-V junction. There is normally a minimal delay between sinus node impulse formation and the beginning of P wave inscription on the electrocardiogram. If this "bridge" (the S-A junction) be-comes diseased, block in the S-A junction may occur.

First-degree S-A block cannot be recognized clinically because there is no effect on the absolute or relative pattern of P waves and QRS complexes; and, of course, the sinus node impulse does not appear on the clinical electrocardiogram.

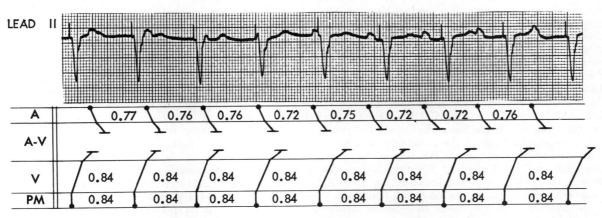

FIG. 131. Complete heart block with a permanent implanted artificial pacemaker. Each QRS complex is preceded by a sharp upright spike which is very narrow and occurs about .02 to .03 second before the QRS. This spike is caused by the artificial pacemaker activity and is called the *pacemaker artifact*. The R-R intervals are precisely .84 second, giving a rate of 71 beats per minute. Other than the presence of the pacemaker artifact and the rate, the tracing fulfills the criteria for complete heart block.

FIG. 132. Second-degree S-A block, Wenckebach type. The QRS complexes and P-R intervals are normal, so that it is immediately evident that the ventricles are discharged by an impulse from above conducted through the A-V node. The P waves are normal in contour; so a sinus mechanism may be assumed. However, there is some irregularity of the P-P intervals which does not demonstrate the smooth slowing and speeding up of a sinus arrhythmia. There is also some group beating evident. Looking now at the group of three complexes in the middle of the tracing, it is evident that the interval between the first two P waves in the group is longer (.63 second) than the interval between the second and third P waves in the group (.60 second). A pause then occurs and the length of the pause is less than twice the P-P interval between the second and third beat (pause = 1.09 seconds, whereas $2 \times .60 = 1.20$ seconds). Thus, these P waves are behaving in the same manner as the QRS complexes in a typical A-V Wenckebach period, i.e., the complexes below the area of the block. With this clue, one should think of the possibility of a Wenckebach type of block *above* the P waves in this group of beats, i.e., in the S-A junction. Since the sinus node impulse formation itself is not indicated on the electrocardiogram, further investigation of this hypothesis must be by indirect evidence. Since the impulse above the area of block in a Wenckebach phenomenon is normal and occurs one more time in any period than the complex below it (because of the dropped beat), it is assumed that in this period of the three P waves there are four sinus node impulses generated, the last being nonconducted. Thus the interval between the first P wave in the group and the first P wave after the pause is measured and divided into four parts (2.32 seconds ÷ 4 = .58 second). We do not know precisely how long before the onset of the first P wave the sinus impulse occurs; therefore we choose an arbitrary value (say .08 second) and call it x. Now measuring .58 second from that point we find that the interval between the time of impulse formation of the second impulse and the second P wave is $x + .05$ second, or an increment of .05 second. The next interval between site of impulse formation and onset of P wave is $x + .07$ second, or an increment of .02 second. There is no P wave following the next sinus node impulse (blocked) and the following sinus impulse falls x second before the first P wave following the pause. Putting all these observations together, we have a lengthening S-A interval with the *increment* of lengthening decreasing (.05 → .02 second), a pause less than twice the P-P interval of the last cycle before the pause, and progressive shortening of the P-P intervals before the pause (.63 → .60 second). These features are exactly analogous to a 4:3 Wenckebach phenomenon in the A-V node. Note also on this tracing the 3:2 period preceding the group of three beats and the intermittent 2:1 S-A block at the end of the tracing.

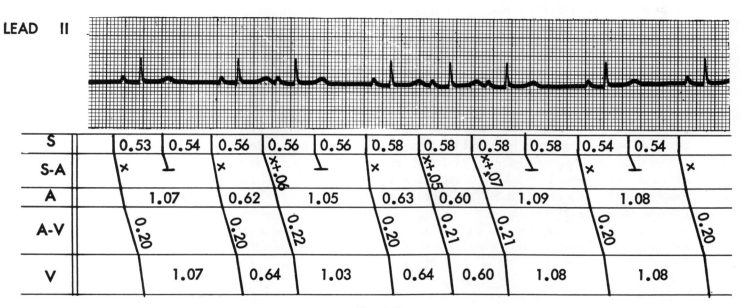

LEAD II

S		0.53	0.54	0.56	0.56	0.56	0.58	0.58	0.58	0.58	0.54	0.54	
S-A		✗	⊥	✗	✗+.06	⊥	✗	✗+.05	✗+.07	⊥	✗	⊥	✗
A		1.07		0.62		1.05		0.63	0.60		1.09		1.08
A-V		0.20		0.20	0.22			0.20	0.21	0.21		0.20		0.20
V			1.07		0.64		1.03		0.64	0.60		1.08		1.08

Fig. 132

285

Second-degree S-A block may be recognized by inference under certain circumstances. For example, *S-A Wenckebach phenomenon* is recognizable because the same Wenckebach manifestations seen below the level of block in A-V nodal Wenckebach (i.e., the effect on the R-R intervals) are seen below the level of block in S-A junction Wenckebach (i.e., the effect on the P-P intervals). Thus, S-A Wenckebach phenomenon is characterized by progressive *shortening* of the P-P intervals, followed by a pause, with a duration less than twice the last or shortest cycle in the period (fig. 132). Since the A-V junction is not involved in S-A Wenckebach phenomenon, the QRS complexes maintain normal relationship to the P waves with a constant P-R interval. Therefore, the R-R interval pattern of variation matches that of the P-P intervals.

The intermittent type of second-degree S-A block is manifested by dropped P waves, just as intermittent second-degree A-V block is manifested by dropped QRS complexes. However, when it occurs in a fixed form, such as constant 2:1, 3:1, 4:1, it is unrecognizable in the clinical electrocardiogram because the rhythm remains constant. But when the block is irregularly intermittent (fig. 133), a pause occurs which bears a whole-number relationship to the sinus cycle and is therefore recognizable. A long pause, not related numerically (as a multiple of the sinus rate) to the sinus cycle length, is referred to as sinus pause or sinus arrest, rather than S-A block.

Third-degree, or complete, S-A block is not recognizable clinically.

In summary, for S-A block to be identifiable on the clinical electrocradiogram, it must be of the Wenckebach type or of the intermittent type of second-degree block (type II).

Special Terms Used to Describe Block. So far, we have been discussing only block of the forward-conducted impulse (that is, block of the impulse originating above and moving toward the ventricles), or *anterograde block*. Conversely, when a primary pacemaker of the heart is present at a junctional or ventricular level (as in junctional or ventricular tachycardia), block in the reverse direction—or *retrograde block* from ventricle or A-V node to atria, across the A-V junc-

286

tion—may occur. The cases in which block in one direction is absent while block in the other direction is present demonstrates that *unidirectional block* may occur. It is a complex and poorly understood pathophysiological phenomenon. The concept of unidirectional block is very important in the understanding of reciprocal rhythm (Chapter 18).

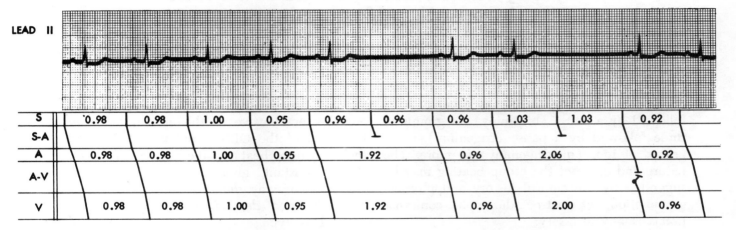

S	0.98	0.98	1.00	0.95	0.96	0.96	0.96	1.03	1.03	0.92
S-A										
A	0.98	0.98	1.00	0.95	1.92		0.96	2.06		0.92
A-V										
V	0.98	0.98	1.00	0.95	1.92		0.96	2.00		0.96

LEAD II

Fig. 133. Intermittent second-degree sinoatrial (S-A) block (type II). The first five complexes on the tracing are normal sinus beats at a rate of approximately 60 per minute. This is followed by a pause approximately equal to two cycle lengths. No P wave is seen during this pause. Since the pause is equal to two cycle lengths, it is inferred that the normal pacemaker function of the sinus node has not been interrupted and that the block, therefore, must have occurred between the sinus node and the atrial tissue (S-A junction). The second pause (between the seventh and eighth beats) is terminated by a junctional escape beat, because this pause is long enough to allow escape of the intrinsic junctional pacemaker. The clue to the escape mechanism is the short *P-R* interval of the eighth beat, indicating that the A-V node escaped before the atrial impulse could be conducted through the A-V node.

CHAPTER EIGHTEEN

Dysrhythmic Patterns Due to Various Interacting Mechanisms

Group Beating. It is frequently possible to identify a regular or recurring pattern of beating in an arrhythmia. Beats may occur in pairs followed by a pause (bigeminy), in groups of three followed by a pause (trigeminy), or in groups of four (quadrigeminy) or more. The nature and cause of the group beating may be suggested by the clinical history and physical examination, but electrocardiographic confirmation is usually necessary.

The most common causes of bigeminal rhythm are premature atrial (fig. 134) or premature ventricular (fig. 135) beats. The electrocardiogram is characterized by a normal sinus beat followed closely by an early atrial or an early ventricular beat. The group is followed by a noncompensatory pause after a premature atrial

beat or by a fully compensatory pause after a premature ventricular beat. The coupling interval (i.e., the time between the onset of the QRS complex or P wave of the normal beat and the onset of the QRS complex or P wave of the premature beat) in these types of bigeminy is constant, giving rise to the concept that in some way *the premature beat is triggered by and dependent upon the normal beat.* This type of premature beat only occurs after the beat to which it is coupled and does not occur during a pause. Various theories proposed to explain this relationship are summarized by Katz and Pick and by Massie and Walsh.

Bigeminy may occur between any two pacemakers. Thus, there may be sinus-ventricular bigeminy, sinus-atrial bigeminy (commonly called atrial bigeminy), ventricular-ventricular bigeminy (i.e., bigeminy due to two separate ventricular foci, one being the primary pace-maker of the heart and the other being the coupled focus), nodal-ventricular bigeminy (A-V nodal primary pacemaker and ventricular ectopic), and other combinations.

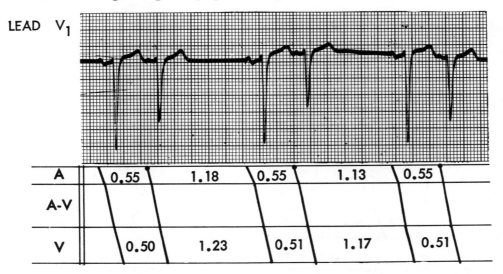

LEAD V₁

A	0.55	1.18	0.55	1.13	0.55
A-V					
V	0.50	1.23	0.51	1.17	0.51

FIG. 134. Atrial bigeminy. The first, third, and fifth P-QRS complexes on the tracing are normal sinus beats. Each is followed by a premature atrial beat with slightly aberrant conduction, and there is a pause after each premature beat. Therefore, the characteristic feature is groups of two beats—one normal and one premature—followed by a pause.

The *coupling interval*, the interval between the sinus P wave and the ectopic P wave, is constant at .55 second. The pattern is designated as *atrial* bigeminy because the coupled ectopic beats are atrial in origin.

Trigeminy is the occurrence of beats in groups of three. It may present as two sinus beats followed by one ectopic beat or as one sinus beat followed by two consecutive ectopic beats. The subsequent pause causes the pattern of the triple rhythm.

Any group beating may be caused by *conduction disturbances (especially the Wencke-*

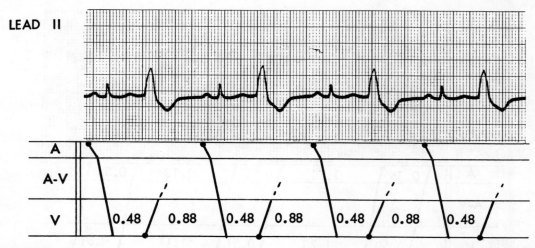

LEAD II

FIG. 135. Ventricular bigeminy. The first, third, fifth, and seventh complexes on the electrocardiogram are normal sinus beats. Each of these is followed by an ectopic beat of abnormal configuration and prolongation beyond .12 second. No P waves precede these ectopic beats. (Note: The positive deflections preceding the ectopic beats are the T waves of the preceding sinus beats.) The ectopic beats are coupled to the preceding sinus beats by a *fixed coupling interval* of .48 second, as measured from the onset of the sinus QRS to the onset of the ectopic QRS. A pause then occurs, and therefore the beats are occurring in groups of two, or bigeminy. Since the ectopic beats fulfill the criteria for *ventricular ectopic beats* and since the pattern is groups of two beats, the rhythm is called *ventricular bigeminy.*

290

bach phenomenon), without any ectopic activity occurring. For example, a 3:2 Wenckebach phenomenon will produce perceptible bigeminy of the pulse and a 4:3 Wenckebach will produce trigeminy. These are easy to differentiate from ventricular bigeminy and trigeminy on the electrocardiogram and sometimes may be distinguished clinically as well.

The Parasystoles. Parasystole is characterized by a primary cardiac pacemaker and another automatic pacemaker which is *independent* of the primary pacemaker (i.e., one is not required to trigger the other as is the case with ectopic beats with fixed coupling intervals). The most common form of parasystole is *ventricular parasystole.* In this arrhythmia, a sinus node pacemaker drives the heart, while a second automatic pacemaker in the ventricles (which is protected from, and thus not discharged by, the descending sinus impulse because of a form of block) is intermittently discharging the ventricles (fig. 136). The ventricular pacemaker is normally slower than the sinus pacemaker. When the ventricular pacemaker is faster it usurps the primary function of the heart and a ventricular tachycardia results.

The electrocardiographic features of ventricular parasystole are *ventricular ectopic beats not coupled to the preceding sinus beats by fixed intervals* (i.e., the interval between the onset of the preceding sinus QRS and the onset of the parasystolic QRS is *not constant*) and showing no fixed pattern of variability. The *parasystolic complexes are related to each other* in a definite mathematical relationship. The interectopic interval (from the onset of one ectopic QRS to the onset of the next) is a multiple of a common denominator, as demonstrated in fig. 136. Whenever the parasystolic impulse occurs while the ventricles are still refractory from the previous beat, the parasystolic focus does not discharge the ventricles and the automatic beat does not occur. If an automatic beat fails to occur following an impulse outside of the refractory period of the previous beat, however, *exit block* is proposed. Exit block is a form of conduction disturbance, rather than a physiological refractoriness, and it prevents the automatic impulse from exiting form its site of origin.

FIG. 136. Ventricular parasystole. Three leads from an electrocardiogram demonstrating ventricular parasystole are shown. The basic mechanism is a normal sinus rhythm. However, numerous ventricular extrasystoles are present.

The coupling interval between the normal sinus beats and the extrasystoles is studied first. If the extrasystoles were the ordinary type of dependent premature ventricular beats (as demonstrated in Chapter 15, figs. 117 and 118; and in this chapter, fig. 135), the coupling interval between the extrasystole and the normal sinus beat preceding it would tend to be constant. However, on this tracing, the coupling intervals are variable and range from .44 (first extrasystole in Lead III) to .60 second (between the seventh and eighth complexes in Lead III). If the coupling intervals of the three fusion beats (third complex on Lead II, fourth complex on Lead III, and last complex on Lead aV_F) are included, the range of coupling intervals is extended to .44 to 1.12 seconds. The presence of *variable coupling intervals* and *fusion beats* is strong evidence for the presence of parasystole.

Next, the *interectopic intervals* are studied. The purpose of this is to determine the frequency of discharge of the ectopic pacemaker and to demonstrate that it is relatively constant. It should also demonstrate that the ectopic discharge depolarizes the ventricles whenever they are not refractory. The frequency of ectopic impulse formation should be independent of the rate of sinus impulse formation. Note that the sinus rate is somewhat variable in the range of 75 to 80 per minute. The interectopic intervals on the tracing should be care-fully measured, since a common denominator of these intervals can be calculated to determine the rate of the automatic ectopic pacemaker. This tracing is particularly simple in this regard because automatic beats are occurring in pairs at several places, and this gives the ectopic frequency directly. Thus, in Lead II, the interval between the seventh and eighth, between the eighth and ninth, and between the last two complexes on the tracing is .94 second. This makes the automatic rate 64 impulses per minute. Note that the interval between the second complex in Lead II (ectopic beat) and the third complex (fusion beat) is also .94 second. If the pairs of ectopic beats were not present (as frequently happens), the ectopic pacemaker rate could be determined in another way. When the intervals between nonpaired ectopic beats are measured, a series of numbers which have common denominators is obtained. For instance, in Lead II, the interval between the third complex (fusion beat) and the seventh complex (ectopic beat) is 2.80 seconds; the interval between the ninth complex and the fourteenth complex is 3.72 seconds. Therefore, since 2.80 seconds is approximately $3 \times .93$ second and 3.72 seconds is $4 \times .93$ second, the largest common denominator is .93 second. Calculating through the rest of the tracing in this manner, the common denominator remains in the range of .93 to .95 second.

If .94 second is measured from the onset of the third complex in Lead II, it becomes evident that the next ectopic impulse falls in the refractory period of the fourth complex and does not, therefore, discharge the ventricles. The same holds true for the next ectopic impulse. But the one following the latter falls beyond the

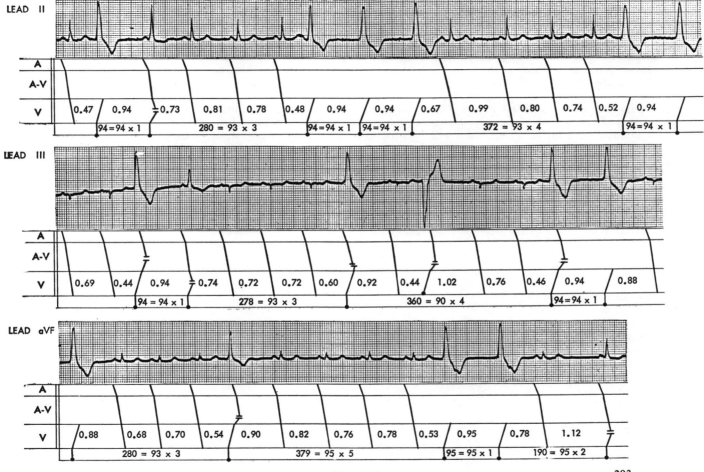

FIG. 136

293

refractory period and discharges the ventricles. The shortest coupling interval on the tracing is .44 second (between the second and third complexes in Lead III). This appears to be the shortest time from the onset of the QRS of a normal sinus complex in which an ectopic impulse can discharge the ventricles. Using this critical interval of .44 second, it should be demonstrable that no impulse occurring earlier than this will discharge the ventricles and no impulse occurring later than this will fail to discharge the ventricles.

The tenth complex on Lead III is a premature beat from another focus and is not part of the parasystolic mechanism.

In summary, this electrocardiogram demonstrates a normal sinus rhythm at a rate of about 75 to 80 per minute, interrupted by a second, automatic focus of impulse formation firing at a rate of about 64 per minute. The secondary focus discharges the ventricles whenever they are not refractory from the primary focus. The ectopic beats do not show fixed coupling to the sinus beats preceding them, and several fusion beats are present.

Ventricular parasystole is the most common form of parasystole, but parasystole may occur between the sinus pacemaker and an ectopic atrial focus (fig. 137) or the sinus pacemaker and an ectopic A-V nodal focus or, very rarely, between any other two automatic centers, one being the primary pacemaker of the heart and the other the parasystolic pacemaker.

Fusion Beats. When two pacemakers discharge at such time that each is able to depolarize part of the ventricular musculature before they physiologically interfere with each other, a ventricular *fusion beat* results. Electrocardiographically, the fusion QRS-T complex is intermediate in contour between the configuration of the QRS complexes of each of the pacemakers (fig. 138). The two foci can often be demonstrated to discharge very closely to ach other. Atrial fusion beats also occur by the same mechanisms as ventricular fusion beats. Fusion beats are common in parasystoles.

Reciprocal Rhythm. A reciprocal ventricular beat is a QRS complex which is caused by an impulse that originates in the ventricle, or A-V junction, leaves it, and then returns to discharge

it a second time. The impulse from the original ventricular beat travels retrogradely through part of the A-V junction. Upon reaching the junction between atria and A-V node, the impulse enters another part of the A-V junction anterogradely to discharge the ventricles once again (fig. 139). Two unusual pathophysiological states are proposed to explain reciprocal rhythm: (1) unidirectional block and (2) longitudinal dissociation in the A-V junction. In unidirectional block, conducting tissue is able to function in one direction but not in the other; and longitudinal dissociation means that an impulse can pass through one part of the A-V junction without affecting another part (Katz and Pick). Thus, in reciprocal rhythm, one part of the A-V junction conducts the retrograde impulse and the other part blocks the impulse (unidirectional block).

While the part with retrograde block is able to conduct anterogradely, the longitudinal dissociation "insulates" that part from the passing impulse, and the impulse does not enter until it reaches the top of the A-V junction. Then it enters that part of the junction

FIG. 137. Atrial parasystole. In atrial parasystole, as in ventricular parasystole, two independent foci are competing. In this case, however, both sites of impulse formation are supraventricular. Therefore, the QRS complexes are of the same configuration whether they are due to ectopic focus discharge or to sinus node discharge.

Varying coupling intervals are again characteristic, as are *fusion beats;* but in atrial parasystole, the fusion beats are atrial fusions (P waves) rather than ventricular. Note that there are three P wave configurations present on the tracing: (1) the short P waves of sinus node origin as in the first complexes in both leads; (2) the tall P waves of ectopic origin as in the third complexes of both leads; and (3) the P waves of intermediate configuration (fusion beats) as in the ninth complex on Lead II and the twelfth complex on Lead V-1.

The coupling intervals vary from .36 (from the onset of the tenth P wave on Lead II to the onset of the eleventh P wave) to .66 second (between the eleventh and twelfth P waves on Lead V-1).

The shortest interectopic interval is 1.02 seconds. All other interectopic intervals are approximate whole-number multiples of 1.01 to 1.02 seconds. Thus, the independent ectopic rate of impulse formation is about 60 per minute. The sinus rate is about 90 per minute. (See fig. 136 for method of calculation of independent ectopic discharge rate.)

In summary, there is a sinus mechanism at a rate of 90 per minute interrupted by an independent ectopic mechanism at a rate of 60 per minute. The independent ectopic impulse discharges the atria anytime that it occurs .36 second or more beyond the onset of the preceding sinus P wave.

296

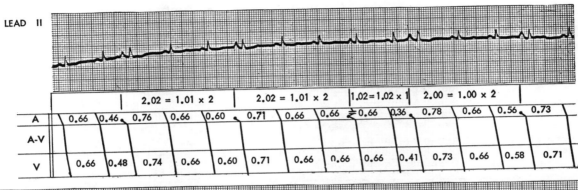

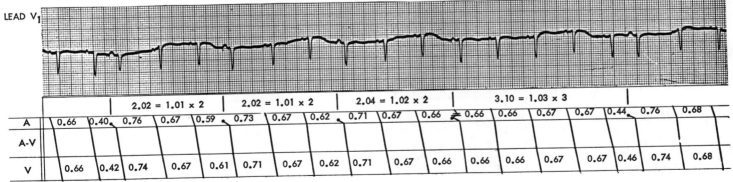

Fig. 137

and reenters the ventricular conducting system.

The electrocardiogram reveals an ectopic A-V nodal or ventricular beat followed by an inverted P wave, which is in turn followed by a normal (anterograde) QRS complex.

Reciprocal atrial beats also occur, but they are very rare and often difficult to identify with any degree of certainty.

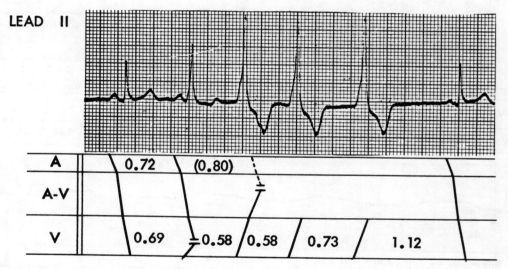

FIG. 138. Fusion beat. The first and last beats on the tracing are normal sinus beats. The third, fourth, and fifth beats are of ventricular origin. Note, however, the second beat. It is intermediate between the first and third beat in (1) voltage, (2) QRS duration, (3) QRS configuration, and (4) T wave configuration. In addition, the R-R interval between it and the third beat is the same as between the third and fourth beat. Finally, the P-R interval of the fusion beat is shorter than the P-R intervals of the sinus beats—a phenomenon which may also occur with fusion.

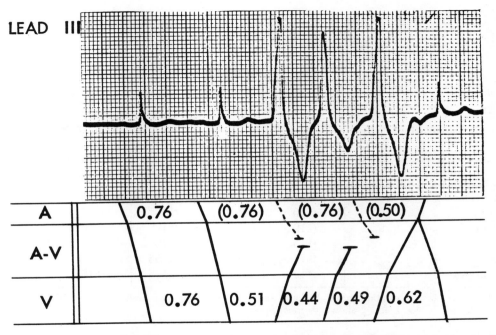

LEAD III

A	0.76	(0.76)	(0.76)	(0.50)
A-V				
V	0.76	0.51	0.44	0.49	0.62

FIG. 139. Reciprocal beat. The last beat of ventricular origin on the tracing (fifth QRS complex) is followed by an inverted P wave (at the end of the T wave). The inverted P wave is then coupled to a normal QRS complex by a P-R interval of about .22 second. As shown in the A-V diagram, the impulse originates in the ventricles and is conducted retrogradely through the A-V junction. It then discharges the atria retrogradely, as well as re-enters the A-V junction to discharge the ventricles again.

Appendix

Table 1 *

UPPER LIMITS OF THE NORMAL P-R INTERVALS (DURATION IN SECONDS)

(From Ashman and Hull)

Rate	Below 70	71–90	91–110	111–130	Above 130
Large adults	0.21	0.20	0.19	0.18	0.17
Small adults	0.20	0.19	0.18	0.17	0.16
Children, ages 14–17	0.19	0.18	0.17	0.16	0.15
Children, ages 7–13	0.18	0.17	0.16	0.15	0.14
Children, ages 1½–6	0.17	0.165	0.155	0.145	0.135
Children, ages 0–1½	0.16	0.15	0.145	0.135	0.125

*The authors express appreciation to Dr. Richard Ashman, Dr. Edgar Hull, and The Macmillan Company for permitting us to use Tables 1 and 2 shown in the Appendix.

*Table 2 **

NORMAL Q-T INTERVALS AND THE UPPER LIMITS OF THE NORMAL
(From Ashman and Hull)

Cycle lengths, sec.	Heart rate per min.	Men and children, sec.	Women, sec.	Upper limits of normal Men and children, sec.	Women, sec.
1.50	40.0	0.449	0.461	0.491	0.503
1.40	43.0	0.438	0.450	0.479	0.491
1.30	46.0	0.426	0.438	0.466	0.478
1.25	48.0	0.420	0.432	0.460	0.471
1.20	50.0	0.414	0.425	0.453	0.464
1.15	52.0	0.407	0.418	0.445	0.456
1.10	54.5	0.400	0.411	0.438	0.449
1.05	57.0	0.393	0.404	0.430	0.441
1.00	60.0	0.386	0.396	0.422	0.432
0.95	63.0	0.378	0.388	0.413	0.423
0.90	66.5	0.370	0.380	0.404	0.414
0.85	70.5	0.361	0.371	0.395	0.405
0.80	75.0	0.352	0.362	0.384	0.394
0.75	80.0	0.342	0.352	0.374	0.384
0.70	86.0	0.332	0.341	0.363	0.372
0.65	92.0	0.321	0.330	0.351	0.360
0.60	100.0	0.310	0.318	0.338	0.347
0.55	109.0	0.297	0.305	0.325	0.333
0.50	120.0	0.283	0.291	0.310	0.317
0.45	133.0	0.268	0.276	0.294	0.301
0.40	150.0	0.252	0.258	0.275	0.282
0.35	172.0	0.234	0.240	0.255	0.262

*The authors express appreciation to Dr. Richard Ashman, Dr. Edgar Hull, and The Macmillan Company for permitting us to use Tables 1 and 2 shown in the Appendix.

Table 3

INTERVAL-RATE CHART

Interval, sec.	Rate, beats per min.	Interval, sec.	Rate, beats per min.
0.20	300	0.70	86
0.22	273	0.72	83
0.24	250	0.74	81
0.26	231	0.76	79
0.28	214	0.78	77
0.30	200	0.80	75
0.32	188	0.82	73
0.34	176	0.84	71
0.36	167	0.86	70
0.38	158	0.88	68
0.40	150	0.90	67
0.42	143	0.92	65
0.44	136	0.94	64
0.46	130	0.96	63
0.48	125	0.98	61
0.50	120	1.00	60
0.52	115	1.02	59
0.54	111	1.04	58
0.56	107	1.06	57
0.58	103	1.08	56
0.60	100	1.10	55
0.62	97	1.12	54
0.64	94	1.14	53
0.66	91	1.16	52
0.68	88	1.18	51

Table 3 (cont.)

Interval, sec.	Rate, beats per min.	Interval, sec.	Rate, beats per min.
1.20	50	1.60	38
1.22	49	1.62	37
1.24	48	1.64	37
1.26	48	1.66	36
1.28	47	1.68	36
1.30	46	1.70	35
1.32	45	1.72	35
1.34	45	1.74	34
1.36	44	1.76	34
1.38	43	1.78	34
1.40	43	1.80	33
1.42	42	1.82	33
1.44	42	1.84	33
1.46	41	1.86	32
1.48	41	1.88	32
1.50	40	1.90	32
1.52	39	1.92	31
1.54	39	1.94	31
1.56	38	1.96	31
1.58	38	1.98	30
		2.00	30

Glossary

Aberrant conduction An abnormal pathway of conduction through the heart due to physiologic refractoriness of part of the conducting system.

Anterograde conduction Conduction in the normal, forward pathway between the sinus node and ventricular myocardium.

Arrhythmia An abnormality or variation of the cardiac rhythm.

Automaticity The property of the heart responsible for impulse formation.

A-V diagram A horizontal line diagram used to graphically demonstrate rhythm events.

A-V dissociation Independent activity of the atria and ventricles.

A-V junction The specialized tissue forming the electrical "bridge" of conduction between the atria and ventricles, and largely responsible for the normal delay between atrial depolarization and ventricular depolarization.

Bifascicular block Block of the right bundle branch plus one of the divisions of the left bundle branch.

Bigeminy Beats occurring in pairs.

Block A pathologic state in the conducting system causing the propagation of an impulse to be slowed or stopped.

Bradycardia A heart rate of less than 60 beats per minute.

Bundle branch block A delay or block of conduction in the left or right branch of the bundle of His.

Conduction The property of impulse transmission.

Coupling interval The interval between a sinus beat and a premature beat, or between any two beats occurring in pairs.

Delta wave Initial QRS wave of slow depolarization due to a bypass tract.

Ectopic beat A beat caused by an impulse originating in an area other than the sinus node.

Escape beat A beat originating in one of the lower pacemaker centers of the heart with a slower intrinsic rate—due to failure of the faster sinus node pacemaker to discharge.

Extrasystole See "Premature beat."

Fibrillation Uncoordinated, irregular activity of cardiac muscle, ineffective for pumping blood.

Fusion beat A complex intermediate in configuration between complexes of two different origins, due to

304

simultaneous discharge of parts of the myocardium by each of the two sites of impulse formation.

Hemiblock   Block in one of the divisions of the left bundle branch.

Hypertrophy   Enlargement due to increase in mass.

Interference   Two impulses traveling toward each other from different directions and preventing each other's passage.

Interpolated beat   An extra beat occurring between two sinus beats without affecting the sinus cycle *or* ventricular cycle.

Interval   The time between two electrocardiographic events.

Intrinsic pacemaker rate   The rate at which a pacemaker focus spontaneously discharges.

Inverted wave   A complex (especially P waves or T waves) whose major deflection is opposite in direction to what would be expected normally in a given lead.

Myocardial infarction   The death of cardiac muscle due to anoxia.

P wave   The electrocardiographic representation of atrial depolarization.

Pacemaker cells   Those specialized cells responsible for the initiation of a cardiac impulse.

Parasystole   A rhythm in which the heart is being paced by two independent pacemakers.

Paroxysmal tachycardia   A tachycardia of sudden onset and sudden end.

Pause   A delay between consecutive impulses.

Pericarditis   An inflammation of the pericardium surrounding the heart.

Potential   The difference in electrical charge between two points, as between the inside and outside of a cell.

P-P interval   The period of time between the onset of one P wave and the onset of the next P wave.

P-R interval   The duration of time between the onset of the P wave (atrial depolarization) and the onset of the QRS complex (ventricular depolarization).

Pre-excitation   Early activation of a portion of the ventricles due to the presence of a bypass tract.

Premature beat   An early beat not in the normal sequence of cardiac impulses.

Purkinje network   The terminal ramifications of the conducting system in the ventricular myocardium.

QRS complex   The electrocardiographic representation of ventricular depolarization.

QRS loop   The sequential connection of the instantaneous vectors of ventricular depolarization.

QRS-T angle   The angle between the mean QRS vector and the mean T wave vector.

Q-T interval   The duration of time between the onset of the QRS complex (ventricular depolarization) and the end of the T wave (ventricular repolarization).

Reciprocal beat   A complex triggered by an impulse which has left and then reentered its area of origin.

Refractory period, absolute   The period of the cardiac

electrical cycle after a discharge, during which the electrically active tissue cannot transmit, or respond to, an impulse.

Refractory period, relative That period of the cardiac electrical cycle after the absolute refractory period, during which the electrically active tissue can transmit, or respond to, an impulse only to a subnormal extent.

Repolarization The recharging of the cell membrane which has been discharged or depolarized.

Resting transmembrane potential The potential across the cell membrane of an electrically active cell when it is fully charged and resting.

Retrograde conduction Conduction backward in the conducting system along a pathway from the ventricles or the A-V node to the atria.

R-P interval The period of time between the onset of a QRS complex and the onset of the following P wave.

R-R interval The period of time between the onset of one QRS complex and the onset of the next QRS complex.

S-A junction The physiologic "bridge" between the site of impulse formation in the sinus node and the atrial myocardium.

Spontaneous depolarization The slow, automatic depolarization of a pacemaker cell, critical in impulse formation.

ST segment The portion of the ECG between the end of the QRS complex and the beginning of the T wave.

Standstill, cardiac The complete cessation of electrical and mechanical activity of the heart.

Supraventricular Pertaining to a beat, or run of beats, whose site of impulse formation is above the ventricular level.

T wave The electrocardiographic representation of ventricular repolarization.

Ta wave The atrial T wave; the wave of repolarization associated with the P wave.

Tachycardia A heart rate of greater than 100 beats per minute.

Trifascicular block Block in the right bundle branch, one division of the left bundle branch, and delayed conduction in the second division of the left bundle branch.

Trigeminy Beats occurring in groups of three.

U wave A deflection which is of uncertain origin, which is not always evident, and which follows the T wave when it is visible.

Vector, electrocardiographic The representation of the direction in space and the magnitude of the electrical activity of the heart.

Vector, instantaneous The spatial direction and magnitude of an electrocardiographic representation of a cardiac electrical event at an instantaneous point in time.

Vector, mean The average direction and magnitude of an electrocardiographic representation of a cardiac electrical event (e.g., mean QRS vector, mean T wave vector).

Bibliography

Part One

ASHMAN, R., BYER, E., and BAYLEY, R. H.: The normal human ventricular gradient; factors which affect its direction and its relation to the mean QRS axis, with an appendix on notation, *Am. Heart J.*, **25**:16, 1943.

BAYLEY, R. H.: An interpretation of the injury and the ischemic effects of myocardial infarction in accordance with the laws which determine the flow of electric currents in homogeneous volume conductors, and in accordance with relevant pathologic changes, *Am. Heart J.*, **24**:514, 1942.

BAYLEY, R. H.: On certain applications of modern electrocardiographic theory to the interpretation of electrocardiograms which indicate myocardial disease, *Am. Heart J.*, **26**:769, 1943.

BAYLEY, R. H.: The electrocardiographic effects of injury at the endocardial surface of the left ventricle, *Am. Heart J.*, **31**:677, 1946.

CONWAY, J. P., CRONVICH, J. A., and BURCH, G. E.: Observations on the spatial vectorcardiogram in man, *Am. Heart J.*, **38**:537, 1949.

DONZELOT, E., and MILOVANOVICH, J.-B.: Introduction à la vectorgraphie spatiale et à l'electrocardiographie vectorielle, *Arch. d. mal. du coeur*, **41**:586, 1948.

DUCHOSAL, P. W., and SULZER, R.: "Vectorcardiographie," Karger, Basle, Switzerland, 1949.

DURRER, D., VAN DAM, R. T., FREUD, G. E., JANSE, M. J., MEIJLER, F. S., and ARZBAECHER, R. C.: Total excitation of the isolated human heart, *Circulation*, **41**:899, 1970.

ESTES, E. H.: Electrocardiography and Vectorcardiography, in HURST, J. W., and LOGUE, R. B. (eds.), "The Heart," McGraw-Hill Book Company, New York, 1970, p. 300.

GRANT, R. P.: "Clinical Electrocardiography," McGraw-Hill Book Company, New York, 1957.

GRANT, R. P.: Left axis deviation; an electrocardiographic-pathologic correlation study, *Circulation*, **14:** 233, 1956.

GRANT, R. P.: Spatial vector electrocardiography; a method for calculating the spatial electrical vectors of the heart from conventional leads, *Circulation*, **2:**676, 1950.

GRANT, R. P.: The relationship of unipolar chest leads to the electrical field of the heart, *Circulation*, **1:**878, 1950.

GRANT, R. P., ESTES, E. H., JR., and DOYLE, J. T.: Spatial vector electrocardiography; the clinical characteristics of the ST and T vectors, *Circulation*, **3:**182, 1951.

GRISHMAN, A., BORUN, E. R., and JAFFE, H. L.: Spatial vectorcardiography; technique for the simultaneous recording of the frontal, sagittal, and horizontal projections, I, *Am. Heart J.*, **41:**483, 1951.

LENEGRE, J.: Etiology and pathology of bilateral bundle branch block in relation to complete heart block. *Progr. Cardiovascular Diseases*, **6:**409, 1964.

LEPESCHKIN, E. (ed.): U wave of the electrocardiogram (symposium), *Circulation*, **15:**68, 1957.

LEV, M.: Normal anatomy of the conduction system in man and its pathology in atrioventricular block. *Ann. N.Y. Acad. Sci.*, **111:**817, 1964.

MACRUZ, R., PERLOFF, J. K., and CASE, R. B.: A method for the electrocardiographic recognition of atrial enlargement, *Circulation*, **17:**882, 1958.

MASSIE, E., and WALSH, T. J.: "Clinical Vectorcardiography and Electrocardiography," The Year Book Medical Publishers, Inc., Chicago, 1960.

MORRIS, J. J., ESTES, E. H., WHALEN, R. E., THOMPSON, H. K., and MCINTOSH, H. D.: P wave analysis in valvular heart disease, *Circulation*, **29:**242, 1964.

MYERBURG, R. J., NILSSON, K., and GELBAND, H.: Physiology of canine intraventricular conduction and endocardial excitation, *Circ. Res.*, **30:**217, 1972.

NAHUM, L. H., MAURO, A., CHERNOFF, H. M., and SIKAND, R. S.: Instantaneous equipotential distribution on surface of the human body for various instants in the cardiac cycle, *J. Appl. Physiol.*, **3:**454, 1951.

ROSENBAUM, M. B., ELIZARI, M. V., and LAZZARI, J. O.: Hemiblocks, Oldsmar, Florida, Tampa Tracings, 1970.

SCHAFFER, A. I., DIX, J. H., and BERGMANN, P.: The effect of eccentricity on spatial vector analysis of the electrocardiogram of the newborn infant and on the correlation between the electrocardiogram and the vectorcardiogram, *Am. Heart J.*, **43:**716, 1952.

SCHER, A. M.: Excitation of the heart, in "Handbook of Physiology," sec. 2, Circulation, vol. 1, American Physiological Society, Washington, 1962, p. 287.

SCHLANT, R. C., and HURST, J. W. (eds.): "Advances in Electrocardiography," Grune & Stratton, New York, 1972.

SODI-PALLARES, D., and CALDER, R. M.: "New Bases of Electrocardiography," C. V. Mosby Company, St. Louis, 1956.

WATT, T. B., and PRUITT, R. D.: Electrocardiographic

findings associated with experimental arborization block in dogs. *Am. Heart J.*, **69:**642–654, 1965.

WILSON, F. N., MACLEOD, A. G., and BARKER, P. S.: The T deflection of the electrocardiogram, *Tr. A. Am. Physicians,* **46:**29, 1931.

WOLFF, L.: Anomalous atrioventricular excitation (Wolff-Parkinson-White) syndrome, *Circulation,* **19:**14, 1959.

WOODBURY, J. W.: Cellular electrophysiology of the heart, in "Handbook of Physiology," sec. 2, Circulation, vol. 1, American Physiological Society, Washington, 1962, p. 237.

Part Two

BELLET, S.: "Clinical Disorders of the Heart Beat," Lea and Febiger, Philadelphia, 1971.

CORDAY, E., and IRVING, D. W.: "Disturbances of Heart Rate, Rhythm, and Conduction," W. B. Saunders Company, Philadelphia, 1961.

DAMATO, A. N., LAU, S. H., HELFANT, R. H., STEIN, E., BERKOWITZ, W. D., and COHEN, S. I.: Study of atrioventricular conduction in man using electrode catheter recordings of His bundle activity, *Circulation,* **39:**287, 1969.

DAMATO, A. N., LAU, S. H., HELFANT, R. H., STEIN, E., PATTON, R. D., SCHERLAG, B. J., and BERKOWITZ, W. D.: Study of heart block in man using His bundle recordings, *Circulation,* **39:**297, 1969.

DREIFUS, L. S., LIKOFF, W., and MOYER, J. H. (eds.): "Mechanisms and Therapy of Cardiac Arrhythmias,"

(Hahnemann Symposium), Grune & Stratton, Inc., New York, 1966.

GRANT, R. P.: The mechanism of A-V arrhythmias, *Am. J. Med.,* **20:**334, 1956.

HOFFMAN, B. F.: The genesis of cardiac arrhythmias, *Progr. Cardiovascular Diseases,* **8:**319, 1965–1966.

HOFFMAN, B. F., and CRANEFIELD, P. F.: "Electrophysiology of the Heart," McGraw-Hill Book Company, New York, 1960.

HOFFMAN, B. F., CRANEFIELD, P. F., and STUCKEY, J. H.: Concealed conduction, *Circulation,* **9:**194, 1961.

HOFFMAN, B. F., CRANEFIELD, P. F., and WALLACE, A. G.: Physiological basis of cardiac arrhythmias, *Mod. Conc. Cardiov. Dis.,* **35:**103, 1966.

KATZ, L. N., and PICK, A.: Current status of theories of mechanisms of atrial tachycardias, flutter and fibrillation, *Progr. Cardiovascular Diseases,* **2:**651, 1960.

KATZ, L. N., and PICK, A.: "Clinical Electrocardiography, Part I, The Arrhythmias," Lea and Febiger, Philadelphia, 1956.

KISTIN, A. D.: Problems in the differentiation of ventricular arrhythmia from supraventricular arrhythmia with abnormal QRS, *Progr. Cardiovascular Diseases,* **9:**1, 1966–1967.

LANGENDORF, R., and PICK, A.: Concealed conduction, *Circulation,* **13:**381, 1956.

LANGENDORF, R., PICK, A., and WINTERNITZ, M.: Mechanisms of intermittent ventricular bigeminy, *Circulation,* **11:**422, 1955.

LEWIS, T.: "The Mechanism and Graphic Registration

of the Heart Beat," Shaw and Son, London, 1925.

MARRIOTT, H. J. L., and MENENDEZ, M. M.: A-V dissociation revisited, *Progr. Cardiovascular Diseases*, 8:522, 1965–1966.

MARRIOTT, H. J. L., and MYERBURG, R. J.: Recognition and Treatment of Cardiac Arrhythmias and Conduction Disturbances, in J. W. HURST and R. B. LOGUE (eds.) "The Heart," McGraw-Hill Book Company, New York, 1970.

MARRIOTT, H. J. L., and SANDLER, I. A.: Criteria, old and new, for differentiating between ectopic ventricular beats and aberrant ventricular conduction in the presence of atrial fibrillation, *Progr. Cardiovascular Diseases*, 9:18, 1966–1967.

MARRIOTT, H. J. L., SCHUBART, A. F., and BRADLEY, S. M.: A-V dissociation; a reappraisal, *Am. J. Cardiol.*, 2:586, 1958.

MASSIE, E., and WALSH, T. J.: "Clinical Vectorcardiography and Electrocardiography," The Year Book Medical Publishers, Inc., Chicago, 1960.

MOE, G. K., and MENDEZ, C.: The physiologic basis of reciprocal rhythm, *Progr. Cardiovascular Diseases*, 8:461, 1965–1966.

SCHAMROTH, L.: Genesis and evolution of ectopic ventricular rhythm, *Brit. Heart J.*, 28:244, 1966.

SCHAMROTH, L., and DOVE, E.: The Wenckebach phenomenon in sinoatrial block, *Brit. Heart J.*, 28:350, 1966.

SCHERF, D., and COHEN, J.: "The Atrioventricular Node and Selected Cardiac Arrhythmias," Grune & Stratton, Inc., New York, 1964.

SCHERF, D., and COHEN, J.: Atrioventricular rhythms, *Progr. Cardiovasular Diseases*, 8:499, 1966.

SCHLANT, R. C., and HURST, J. W. (eds.): "Advances in Electrocardiography," Grune & Stratton, Inc., New York, 1972.

WIT, A. L., WEISS, M. B., BERKOWITZ, W. D., ROSEN, K. M., STEINER, C., and DAMATO, A. N.: Patterns of atrioventricular conduction in the human heart, *Circ. Res.*, 27:345, 1970.

INDEX

Q-T interval, 5, 205
after digitalis, 187, 188, 192, 196

R wave, 3
R′ wave, 3
Rate, measurement of, 221, 223
Reciprocal beats, 295, 298, 299
Repolarization, 4, 44
cellular, 217, 218
after digitalis, 187, 188
in left bundle branch block, 163
in left ventricular hypertrophy, 84, 85
normal ST vector and, 44
in right bundle branch block, 156, 157
in right ventricular hypertrophy, 71
(*See also* T vector)
Reversal of R/S ratio, 69
Right bundle branch block, 155–161
depolarization, 155, 156
duration of QRS complexes, 156
etiology of right bundle branch block, 157
mean ST vector in, 157
mean T vector in, 156, 157
and myocardial infarction, 157
QRS-T angle in, 156, 157
terminal .04 vector in, 156
Right ventricular hypertrophy, 69–82
direction of mean spatial ST vector in, 71

Right ventricular hypertrophy:
direction of mean spatial T vector in, 71
duration of QRS complexes in, 70
instantaneous QRS vectors in, 69
magnitude of QRS vectors in, 70
mean QRS vector in, 69
QRS-T angle in, 71

S wave, 3
S_1, S_2, S_3 pattern, 172, 173, 180, 181
depolarization, 172, 173
Sinoatrial (S-A) block, 282–287
Sinus arrhythmia, 231, 232
Sinus bradycardia, 232, 236
Sinus node, 218, 219
Sinus tachycardia, 233, 237, 238, 272, 274
(*See also* Tachycardia)
Spatial leads, 17
ST segment, 4
ST vector:
after digitalis, 188, 189, 196, 197
in left bundle branch block, 164
in left ventricular hypertrophy, 84
in myocardial infarction, 116, 117
normal, 44, 47, 64, 65
in pericarditis, 198–201
after pulmonary embolism, 203–205
in right bundle branch block, 157

$$r = ? = \frac{\text{BEATS}}{\text{MIN.}} \times$$

$$S = 2 \, ^{sq}/_{beat}$$

$$t = 1 \, ^{sq}/_{.20 \, sec.}$$

$$r = \frac{\#\text{beats}}{60 \, sec.} = \frac{\#\text{beats}}{300 \, squares.}$$

$$r = \frac{\Delta B}{\Delta t}$$

$$\Delta B = 1 \, beat$$

$$\Delta t = \# \, sq. \times .2 \, sec/sq.$$

$$r = \frac{1 \, beat}{2 \, sq \times .2 \, sec/sq \times 1 \, min/60 \, sec.} = \frac{300 \, beat}{\Delta t \, (sq).}$$